SAFE COSMETIC SURGERY:

A COMPLETE GUIDE

SAFE COSMETIC SURGERY:

A COMPLETE GUIDE

Dai Davies FRCS
with
Judy Sadgrove

metro

First published in Great Britain in 1996
by Metro Books (an imprint of Metro Publishing Limited),
19 Gerrard Street, London W1V 7LA

Dai Davies and Judy Sadgrove are hereby identified as the
authors of this work in accordance with Section 77 of the
Copyright, Designs and Patents Act 1988.

British Library Cataloguing in Publication Data. A CIP
record of this book is available on request from the British
Library.

ISBN   1 900512 02 5

10 9 8 7 6 5 4 3 2 1

Design and computer page make up by Tony and Penny Mills
Printed in Great Britain by Clays Ltd, St Ives plc
Diagrams by Richard Burgess
Colour plate section designed by Robert Updegraff

The names and professions of all the interviewees
in this book have been changed
to retain confidentiality.

Contents

ACKNOWLEDGEMENTS

With thanks to Chris Kettler, Nicholas J. Lowe, Brent
Tanner, Douglas Harrison, Peter Mason, John Scurr,
Chris Ward, David Harris and Phyl Costello

Foreword

Cosmetic or 'aesthetic' surgery is not new. It has been practised, particularly in Europe, since the early part of the 20th Century. However, there has been a significant increase in the numbers of patients seeking advice about cosmetic surgery in recent years which has produced an explosion in media and public interest. Inevitably the accuracy of written articles and television presentation varies considerably, some being frankly misleading. This, allied with the profusion of advertisements in the back pages of glossy journals promoting the services of 'cosmetic clinics', can make it extremely difficult for an individual patient to find the help which they require. Choosing a skilled and reputable surgeon is crucial to anyone considering cosmetic surgery. There is no substitute for professional recommendation (either from a general practitioner or another specialist) or, failing this, personal recommendation. However, the information contained within this book will provide a background for the layman to assist in making such a choice.

Over the last 20 years or so there have been many advances in plastic and reconstructive surgery which have had significant 'spin-offs' in the field of cosmetic surgery. This is particularly so in the face where the advent of craniofacial surgery has given a much improved understanding of both the structure and workings of the face from which sophisticated 'rejuvenative' operations have evolved. It is now possible, therefore, to tailor operations more closely to an individual's requirements and as techniques become more varied and sophisticated they inevitably become more difficult for a layman to understand.

It must be remembered that cosmetic surgical procedures are often of a major nature and must be considered very carefully before being undertaken. Having cosmetic surgery is not like visiting the hairdressers as some advertisements would have us believe.

Contrary to popular belief, cosmetic surgery is not restricted by social boundaries and is sought by a spectrum of people across society and income groups. This book has been designed to provide information about the techniques available in an honest way which can be easily understood. It will provide a useful background to anybody considering cosmetic surgery.

CHAPTER ONE

Why Cosmetic Surgery?

You don't have to be an ageing movie star to want cosmetic surgery. Large numbers of ordinary people put themselves into the hands of a cosmetic surgeon. Around 65,000 people submitted themselves to the scalpel last year and numbers are soaring every year in Britain and across Europe. In the US, cosmetic surgery is the fastest growing medical speciality and an estimated two to three million people had surgery last year.

Nine out of ten cosmetic operations are thought to be done to reverse the signs of ageing. The Hollywood stars show us just how effectively surgery can stop the clock. But cosmetic surgery isn't just about smoothing wrinkles and tightening sagging flesh. Many people undertake it not to beautify or rejuvenate themselves but simply to make themselves look more normal. Cosmetic surgery can transform life for someone who feels different because of an out-of-the-ordinary feature, such as a big nose, small breasts or an unsightly scar.

Today, cosmetic surgery is much more acceptable, far more widely available and much cheaper than it used to be. However, it's still mostly women who choose to go through with it, because women tend to be judged more on how they look than men. Probably around 90 per cent of operations are carried out on women, but growing numbers of men are taking the plunge and as many as one in five operations in the US are now done on men. Why? Because men can be just as concerned about their appearance as women. This is especially true if their work exposes them to the media. Youthful looks also give men an edge in the competitive world of business.

People whose work depends on their appearance are under particular pressure to enhance or preserve their looks and they may find the decision to have cosmetic surgery a relatively easy one to make. But many of us feel – particularly if we're a bit older – that having an operation to change the way we look is wrong, that it's interfering with nature, pandering to vanity or just plain frivolous. We may feel concerned about the fact that many people in the world don't get enough to eat, yet some of us are prepared to spend a small fortune on a face-lift.

Youthful looks

We're all caught up to some extent in the billion pound beauty industry, buying new clothes, getting our hair coloured and styled and sampling different face creams, cosmetics and perfumes. The only real difference is that cosmetic surgery changes us permanently. Is someone who wants permanent change any more peculiar than someone who spends hours applying make-up in front of the mirror each day?

We may have been told that we should accept our appearance and that we should grow old gracefully. We may shudder at the very idea of a scalpel slicing into flesh, viewing it as self-mutilation. And many women feel morally outraged that their sisters will resort to being cut open in order to look the way men think they should look.

This negative attitude still prevails in Britain, where people who have had cosmetic surgery will rarely admit to it, fearing the charge of vanity. In the US, where it's much more common, some media stars, such as Cher and Roseanne, are upfront about their many operations. Others, like the pop star Michael Jackson, are more controversial. Yet for many ordinary Americans, having cosmetic surgery is simply another form of self-maintenance, much like going to the gym or to therapy.

It's easy for us to tell ourselves that we should accept the way we look. But it's hard to do this in our society, because we live in a culture that reveres good looks. Beauty and youth *mean* happiness and success. That's the equation we see on TV all the time.

Media stars rely on their looks and devote huge amounts of time, money and energy to maintaining them – time, money and energy the rest of us simply can't afford. Countless numbers of these stars – men as well as women – have had cosmetic surgery. Paula Yates has had her breasts enhanced; Cilla Black has had her nose done; Cher is reported to have had dozens of operations to alter her face and body, including the removal of two ribs to emphasise her waist.

This artificial perfection can make the rest of us feel we just don't match up and a feeling of inadequacy can drive people to cosmetic surgery in an unrealistic quest for film-star flawlessness. A small number of people do indeed seem to be almost addicted to surgery – going back for operation after operation to improve their appearance.

But for most of us, the question of whether or not to have cosmetic surgery will come up just once in our lives. Whether or not you would have a face-lift or some other procedure to make yourself look better is a question most people will have asked themselves or discussed with friends at some time or other. Nowadays, many more of us are prepared to say yes – often after several years' thinking about it.

'I don't see rich women chasing eternal youth,' says one Harley Street surgeon. 'Most of my patients are very ordinary. They've saved up to deal with a specific deformity or they want to deal with the facial sagging that affects women earlier than men and erodes their confidence.'

A psychological need

We tend to make snap judgements about other people the minute we set eyes on them. We respond negatively to people with facial disfigurement and we often overlook the elderly altogether. We may imagine that men with flattened noses are ready to pick a fight and we have a tendency to condemn people who are very fat as lazy, slow and greedy. We may think that people whose ears stick out are less intelligent and the police are much more likely to pick up men with scars on their faces.

There has been a lot of research showing how people generally considered to have pleasing looks are more popular, get better jobs and even lighter prison sentences. Those who are considered to look a bit different can easily become isolated, excluded from friendship and sexual relationships. This isolation can start in school and carry on into adult life.

Having a big nose or goblin ears, being fat or simply wearing glasses can condemn a child to a mocking nickname, robbing him or her of self-confidence. Some children end up as adults never allowing themselves to be photographed, be seen in profile or from one side, or going to endless lengths to hide their nose, or whatever it is that bothers them.

'For these people who have become obsessive, cosmetic surgery can have a wonderful effect, better than years of antidepressants or therapy,' says Dr Eileen Bradbury, a psychologist attached to the plastic surgery unit at the Withington Hospital, Manchester, who has published research on the subject. 'A corrective operation makes someone acceptable, the same as everyone else, setting him or her free from all that anxiety and social phobia.'

One study, carried out in Plymouth by consultant plastic surgeon David Harris, compared the feelings of 400 NHS patients having cosmetic surgery on noses, breasts and tummies, or having tattoos removed, before and after their operations. Mr Harris found that before surgery more than 60 per cent felt extremely self-conscious, embarrassed and unattractive. Many tended to avoid social events and had difficulty establishing sexual relationships. After surgery, there was a dramatic improvement in how confident and outgoing they felt.

'My whole life was dominated by my breasts,' says Laura, aged 25. 'They were massive. Whatever I did, like just popping out to buy the paper, attracted attention. Men stared at me all the time. Even when they didn't say anything, they all mentally undressed me and sized me up. Women used to look at me with pity. My breasts were so heavy that I used to get backache. My bras cut into my shoulders. I've still got the grooves.'

Laura went on to antidepressants after three years at college spent camouflaging her appearance with sloppy jumpers and avoiding men. Her parents were so worried about her that they arranged the operation, which Laura says changed her life.

'I found myself arching back at first, with all that weight

gone from in front but, above all, it's a weight gone from my mind. I no longer feel a freak. I enjoy dressing up and shopping for clothes. Men seem much more friendly and the way they look at me suggests interest in the whole of me, not just my breasts. I can stop worrying about my appearance and get on with the real business of living.'

If a surgeon can be convinced that someone is in real psychological distress about a particular feature, such as their nose or breasts, it may be possible to get cosmetic surgery on the NHS. But waiting lists are long.

Nose reshaping is the most common cosmetic operation of all. This is followed by breast surgery (enhancement and reduction) and face-lifts. Breast enhancement was extremely popular in the 1980s, but has declined as a result of the scare about silicone implants. Today, the fastest growing form of cosmetic surgery in the US is liposuction, the vacuum removal of fat.

Of course, some women who undergo cosmetic surgery are in pursuit of beauty, but sheer vanity is rarely the reason why most people put themselves through it, even when it comes to anti-ageing procedures, according to Dr Bradbury.

'Some people make the decision to have a face-lift in mid life after both parents have died. They look in the mirror and believe they look old. They feel young, but they're scared. I'm next, they think.'

A small group of people seek to alter their appearance in order to deal with a trauma, such as sexual abuse. Women who have been abused sometimes want to change a feature that particularly reminds them of their abuser, and which they see reflected in their faces in the mirror each day.

Cosmetic surgery is not always the right answer. Some

people turn to a surgeon when they are going through a crisis in their work or homelife. They hope that by changing their appearance, their life will change for the better. A man may hope that if he looked younger, his business might do better. A woman may imagine that if her breasts were bigger, her unfaithful husband might come back to her. Or someone may simply turn up to consult the surgeon clutching a photo of someone else, saying, 'I want a nose like that.'

These people should be advised against surgery, since people with unrealistic expectations often regret their operation later on. Surgeons also try to screen out the small number of people who forever seek cosmetic surgery because they suffer from a rare psychiatric condition called dysmorphophobia. These people – who look entirely normal – are convinced that they look ugly or misshapen.

Cosmetic surgery for children

Few parents would dispute the wisdom of their child having cosmetic surgery if he or she is marked out by a defect, such as a hare lip, portwine stain or birthmark, or has been left scarred by a burn, scald or other injury. Children who squint are often recommended for eye surgery. This not only corrects their vision but also produces a straight gaze, which has a huge effect on how we all relate to the child.

Most frequently of all, children with prominent ears have them surgically pinned back. Large numbers also undergo teeth straightening; and small children are sometimes given a dose of growth hormone to make them bigger.

More controversially, a handful of children with Down's syndrome are having facial surgery – the idea being that if they looked more 'normal' they'd be treated more normally.

However, with the exception of ear-pinning and correcting deformities, most cosmetic operations are delayed until children have reached adulthood.

Taking the plunge

The decision to have cosmetic surgery is a personal one. It should never be made at the suggestion of others, not well-meaning friends and relatives and certainly not partners. In fact, most people don't want their partner to have cosmetic surgery but, sadly, some people do consult a surgeon because their partner has teased them or intimated, 'I might love you more if you looked different.' Of course, this is the wrong reason for having surgery.

We live in a ruthlessly competitive era in which we're fighting for work. The old and the ugly are the first to be rejected. So there are going to be more and more of us willing to take advantage of whatever the surgeon can offer to improve and maintain our looks. During the 1980s in the US, the number of people who had surgery to remove excess skin and bags around the eyes went up by over a third and face-lifts by a quarter.

Unfortunately, there are no such figures for Britain, where cosmetic surgery is largely unregulated. Yet, whether we approve of it or not, the fact remains that the cosmetic surgeon can now rejig just about any part of us. You dislike it? The surgeon can fix it – from erasing crow's feet and liver spots to extending the length of a penis.

What are the risks?

New techniques mean we don't always need to have a

general anaesthetic, stay in hospital or even submit to the scalpel. We can have thin lips enlarged with injections of collagen and outlined by tiny dots of colour, or have our frown lines temporarily frozen. We can have the fat sucked out of us by liposuction and we can venture into the future with the use of lasers to eradicate wrinkles.

On the other hand, there have been many scare stories connected to, for example, the safety of collagen, liposuction and silicone breast implants. We also know that the results of cosmetic surgery can be variable, as we've all heard stories of operations that have gone horribly wrong, leaving people scarred, with major loss of sensation or even deformed.

Provided it's carried out by a reputable surgeon and anaesthetist, cosmetic surgery is safe. Of course, there's the general anaesthetic, though the risk of dying under it is extremely rare.

Nevertheless, having cosmetic surgery is still a risky business. Every time a surgeon picks up a scalpel there is a possibility of complications. Surgery is an invasive procedure and it can cause severe pain, appalling bruising and permanent scars. Recovery takes a long time.

The pain will ease and the bruises disappear with time, but how well the scars heal and fade cannot be predicted with any accuracy. How completely scars are hidden depends not only on the skill of the surgeon but also on the type of operation. Anyone contemplating a breast reduction, for instance, needs to know that scars may remain visible and nerves may be severed so that repositioned nipples may lose sensitivity.

Most importantly, satisfaction cannot be guaranteed. Surgery may not fulfil expectations. There may be unexpectedly bad scarring. The patient may be dissatisfied with his or her new appearance, or even feel that he or she hardly looks any different after the operation. Or there may be grave disappointment if a person still doesn't get that top job after having had surgery, or the marriage still breaks up.

Should you tell?

If you do decide to have cosmetic surgery, you have to consider whether or not you want other people to know. Most people who have had a cosmetic operation are extremely reluctant to let the world know what they've done. They don't want to be condemned for vanity. They don't want friends to be horrified at how much money they've spent, neither do they want to be told that they should grow old gracefully.

You should certainly discuss your decision with your partner, who may well feel anxious about all the risks of surgery. It's probably worth telling a trusted friend to see how he or she reacts but otherwise, you may find it easiest, in general, to keep your plans to yourself. It's surprising how often someone undergoes cosmetic surgery and no one spots the change – except to express general admiration for how well they look, or what nice clothes they're wearing.

Refinements in technique and new technology are being developed all the time. A good cosmetic surgeon can do incredible things for your looks but you have to find that surgeon. Even then, it's still a case of sitting down and working out whether the benefits of having a particular operation really outweigh all the risks involved.

Cosmetic surgery is a life event, so it's vital that you think long and hard about why you want to have it. Equally important is finding a surgeon you trust who understands exactly what you want and can tell you whether or not that's possible.

Finding a surgeon is not easy, unless you simply respond to one of the many advertisements at the back of magazines and supplements. However, you don't want to end up looking worse than you did to start with. Surgical mistakes are distressing and costly to put right – if that's possible – so it's well worth making every effort to make sure you get the right one.

Remember, though, cosmetic surgery is not a magic wand. It may alter your appearance, and this may change the way you feel about yourself, but it cannot be guaranteed to change your life. That is up to you, not a cosmetic surgeon.

CHAPTER TWO

Lifting the Face and Neck

When we are young, our faces are round, smooth and firm with our skin fitting snugly over fat, muscle and bone. As we get older, our skin becomes thinner and less elastic, bone is lost and muscles supporting the skin gradually lose tone and stretch. Ligaments and connective tissue weaken so that the fat that gives our face a youthful shape slips down towards the jaw.

The most noticeable effect is a sagging, which shows up in deepening grooves from nose to mouth (the nasolabial fold), jowls and a turkey gobble neck, where two vertical bands of skin stand out in the neck. As eyebrows droop, extra skin may cause hoods and bags around the eyes and fine lines will show up where thin skin is attached to the underlying muscle fibres – around the edge of the mouth and the corners of the eyes.

The rate at which this ageing process occurs is largely determined by our genes. If our parents look young for their age, then so will we and we will also look more youthful if we matured late. Those of us with strong wide cheekbones may appear to age more slowly, because there is less fat to slip down to the jaw.

Lifestyle too plays a big part. A high level of fitness, a nutritious diet and low levels of stress keep our skin in prime condition. Inactivity, a poor diet, heavy smoking and drinking, high levels of stress, excessive suntanning, loss of teeth, repeated frowning and other facial habits all contribute to the overall look of our faces, affecting the complexion, skin elasticity, colouring, shape and development of lines, wrinkles, pouches, jowls and broken capillaries.

OPTING FOR A FACE-LIFT

If you find that your face looks tauter and better when you pull up on the skin in front of your ears, then you might decide to have a face-lift. The best candidates for this operation are men and women aged 40 to 60, whose skin is still elastic and whose bone structure is strong and well-defined.

A face-lift can also be successful in older people in their seventies or eighties. But it is being done more and more on younger people who have aged prematurely as a result of exposure to the sun or smoking.

In fact, many surgeons prefer to operate on younger patients, in order to postpone the signs of ageing rather than trying to turn back the clock. It can be awkward facing people after having apparently lost 15 years overnight, which is why so many media stars opt for their first lift at 40 or so, before their age starts to show.

'I had a face-lift seven weeks ago,' says Jane MacIntyre, who's 49, but looks as though she's in her early thirties. 'It was my neck that I really hated. It was all scraggy and looked older than my face. But I also had hoods over my eyes and I thought I looked tired all the time. I was advised to have an extended SMAS face-lift (*see page 30*) and upper eye surgery.

'I wasn't frightened because I had complete faith in my surgeon, but the operation was still a daunting prospect. I was given the general anaesthetic at 1.30pm and I was awake again at 7pm, when my face felt stiff and swollen. I had some tea but I couldn't eat anything and I was very drowsy.

'Next morning, after dozing through the night, I had breakfast, showered and washed my hair. A friend picked me up from hospital and took me home. My face looked awful – as swollen and bruised as if I'd gone ten rounds with Mike Tyson. On each side of my head I had a little cut hidden in my hair above the ear, another right by the ear and a third behind the ear. And I had a cut under my chin and two fine cuts hidden in the lid line above my eyes.

'I felt tired and sore and slept most of the next 48 hours, propped up on pillows and taking strong painkillers and sleeping pills. My head felt like a football. Four days later, I had my stitches out but I still looked pretty bruised and battered and felt very tired, so I didn't go out properly for another couple of days.

'I was back at work two weeks after the operation, although I think now that I would have preferred another week off. I still needed to wear a lot of make-up to conceal the bruises. My face felt stiff and it hurt to bend down. It took a while to settle down but now it only feels sore when it's cold.

'I look great now. All my expectations have been fulfilled. My face is fresher, the hoods on my eyes have gone and my neck is no longer scraggy. I didn't really tell anyone I was getting it done, and when I met some friends recently, all they said was how well I looked and what a nice suit I was wearing!'

How to go about it

Anyone wanting a face-lift needs to find a surgeon they can trust (*see Chapter 14*). Surgery of any kind is a frightening event, and the fact that you have chosen to have your face cut open doesn't make it any less frightening. As in any surgery, there's always the risk of complications after the operation or bad scarring.

In any case, after a face-lift you will look a terrible mess, with bruising and swelling lasting for days and even weeks. Patients feel extremely vulnerable during this period and need lots of reassurance. You must feel able to turn to your surgeon and the nursing team for support. Never forget that if you require further surgery to repair the first operation, you may have to pay for it.

When you first approach your chosen cosmetic surgeon, you will want to ask him or her what can be done for your face. It's also important that you explain exactly which parts of your face you would like to have changed.

For most people, having a face-lift is a one-off event. Simply going to see a surgeon can make you anxious, which means that you may not take in all that is said at the appointment. It's been found that patients only retain about one-third of the information given to them by their doctor at a consultation. So it's important that you are given written details of your options before you leave.

A proper medical history needs to be taken and the surgeon must make a careful examination of your face, taking account of all aspects of it, including any asymmetries. (The human body is asymmetrical in that if it is divided down the middle, neither side of the imaginary dividing line is quite the same – it's easiest to see when you look at your eyes or breasts. Sometimes we start to worry after cosmetic surgery about a lopsidedness that, in fact, was there before.)

Photographs will be taken and another appointment made for a week or so later, when the surgeon may ask you to wear less make-up. Some surgeons use a polaroid camera to take the photos, so they are instantly available, although a polaroid photo can make anyone look like they need a face-lift! You might like to take along some photographs of when you were younger for reference.

At the second consultation, you will work out together with the surgeon what kind of face-lift you need. Everyone has different requirements, which makes each operation unique. You might also decide that you want to enhance your chin (*see page 36*) or your cheekbones with silicone implants, for example, which are inserted on top of the bone (*see page 87*). Other procedures can also be done at the same time as a face-lift, or later, such as a chemical peel (*see page 78*), dermabrasion (*see page 75*), laser treatment (*see page 90*) or extra eyelid surgery (*see page 56*). And there are all sorts of added extras you can choose from to counteract the effects of time and gravity, such as earlobe shortening (*see page 70*), lip enhancement (*see page 63*) and nose and chin contouring (*see page 40*) .

There are no guarantees with a face-lift. Some people have thick oily skin which doesn't move easily or stretch. Others have thin, sun-damaged skin that responds very well. However, a face-lift will not erase superficial wrinkles, such as crow's feet or lipstick-bleed lines around the mouth, and it may have little effect on the nose to mouth grooves or eye area.

'I paid out £7,000 for a complete facial overhaul last year,' says Jean Sutcliffe, who's 67 and recently widowed. 'Now I'm on my own, I'd like to feel more confident about holidaying on my own. But whenever I caught sight of myself all I ever saw were bags under my eyes, deep creases running from my nose to my mouth and lines around my mouth.

'I thought a face-lift would make me look ten years younger, but I was very disappointed. It was a gradual feeling that developed after the healing process. I hoped everyone would be amazed at the change in me, but no one noticed a thing and my friends who knew I'd had cosmetic surgery wondered whether it had been worth the money.

'The bags under my eyes have gone, but there is some lumpiness and puffiness in my cheeks. The nose-to-mouth lines are still there – in fact one side is now worse than the other, which has been slightly improved. And the scars under my chin where the surgeon removed the fat are still bumpy.

'But it's the general impression really. The operation simply hasn't made much difference. I suppose I'm lucky that my surgeon is aware of my disappointment and he's prepared to try and improve my face further. I hope he can, otherwise it was a waste of money – and I'm not rich. I still haven't had that holiday I promised myself.'

THE RIGHT FACE-LIFT FOR YOU

Fashions come and go when it comes to face-lifts and, as advances are made in surgery, refinements in technique are being made all the time. At present, there are six different versions (*see table on page 28*) of the face-lift – or

THE FACE-LIFT

Surgical Procedure	Definition	Indication	Procedure	Complications
Sub-cutaneous lift	simple skin tightening (from a lunch-time tuck to extensive undermining)	the older patient	IV sedation, and local, or general anaesthetic	haematoma, discoloration, scars, ear deformities, lumps under skin; short-term results from mini lift
SMAS lift	pull on deeper layers of tissue	turkey gobble neck	general anaesthetic, 3 weeks' recovery	risk to nerves, bad scars
Extended SMAS lift (deep plane)	lifting SMAS free from cheek ligaments	nose to mouth grooves, jowls, turkey gobble neck	general anaesthetic, 2–3 weeks' recovery	less swelling, more risk to nerves, less risk of haematoma
Composite lift	as above, plus open brow-lift and extensive lower eyelid surgery	as above, plus drooping brow and eye/cheek bags	general anaesthetic, 4–6 hour operation	swelling for up to 6 months, risk to nerves, altered sensation in scalp
Mask lift	lift all facial structures off bone	nose to mouth grooves, eyelids, younger patient, smokers	general anaesthetic	swelling for 6–12 weeks, altered sensation in scalp, radical change in appearance, especially eyes
Endoscopic (keyhole) lift	as above, via small incisions (also in mouth)	as above	general anaesthetic	swelling for 6–8 weeks, not known how long it lasts

A face-lift

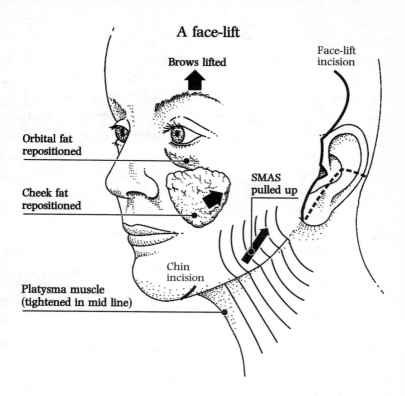

Brows lifted

Face-lift
incision

Orbital fat
repositioned

Cheek fat
repositioned

SMAS
pulled up

Chin
incision

Platysma muscle
(tightened in mid line)

rhytidectomy – and they all have a different impact on the face. It's vital that the surgeon chooses the one that is right for you, rather than simply opting for the one which is currently receiving most publicity.

The mini lift. A basic operation (a subcutaneous lift) in which the surgeon cuts into skin in a line beginning at the temples and running down in front of the ears and behind them across into the scalp. The skin is then lifted up off the facial structures, stretched taut and the excess trimmed off.

This kind of skin-tuck operation can vary from a lunchtime procedure that has little long-term effect to a more extensive undermining of the skin that will prolong recovery. Distortion of the ears often occurs when scars contract and pull them downwards about six months later. The mini lift has no impact on nose-to-mouth grooves, it can leave bad scars behind the ears, in particular, and repeated lifts can create a tight look (usually caused, in fact, by chemical peels carried out in conjunction with the face-lift).

The SMAS face-lift. This is the modern standard operation in which deeper cuts are usually made. The aim is to pull the skin and the SMAS (a layer of tissue and muscle under the skin called the superficial musculo-aponeurotic system) attached to it upwards. Muscles in the lower face and neck are tightened and anchored to bone with stitches where possible. Skin is then redraped over more youthful contours.

Fatty pouches may be removed and implants sometimes added to increase the volume of a narrow face. This operation will improve the appearance of a turkey gobble neck but has little effect on nose-to-mouth grooves. There may be poor scarring and there is a small risk of damage to the facial nerves.

The extended SMAS lift (or deep plane). Burrowing further in towards the nose to lift the SMAS right away from the cheek ligaments and then pulling it up improves the look of the middle of the face, perking up sagging cheeks, flattening nose-to-mouth grooves and reducing jowls, as well as tightening the neck. This operation may produce less swelling than the limited SMAS, fewer scars and recovery can be very quick.

The composite face-lift. A much larger operation, it combines an extended SMAS with a brow-lift (*see page 53*) and lower eyelid surgery so as to treat a drooping brow and eye and cheek bags, as well as the middle and lower face. It is often suitable for the older individual. However, it takes much longer for all the swelling to go down – up to six months – and there is an increased risk of damage to the facial nerves.

The mask lift (or subperiosteal face-lift). This is a new technique which involves both cutting from within the mouth to free the cheeks and tunnelling down from an Alice band incision across the top of the head, under the covering of the bone (periosteum), to move the very deepest layers of fat upwards together with muscle and skin.

The mask lift can have a dramatic effect on appearance, actually changing the way you look by flattening the face a little and giving the eyes a slight Oriental slant. The operation works well on both laughter lines and on the eye area but it produces prolonged swelling, there's a risk of infection in the cheek area, hair may be lost from around the incisions and sensation in the scalp may be permanently altered. In addition, the mask lift is likely to cost much more, simply because it is a new technique that is in vogue.

The endoscopic face-lift. Developments in keyhole (endoscopic) surgery mean that the mask lift, which tends to be recommended for younger patients, can now be carried out through five very small radial incisions in the scalp and via the lower eyelids, without making any cuts inside the mouth.

A fibreoptic light and endoscopic camera is fed through

one scalp incision, so the surgeon can see what he or she is doing on a TV monitor. Through another incision is fed a long-handled instrument, like a curved chisel, which dissects beneath the covering of the bone to avoid damage to the nerves and other structures.

The endoscopic mask lift is an entirely new procedure. So surgeons do not yet know how long the results last. The technique is still being evaluated and refined. Not all cosmetic surgeons are trained to carry out endoscopic surgery and not all hospitals have the equipment, which is being improved all the time.

The endoscopic lift is not less invasive than the ordinary mask lift, the operation is simply carried out through tiny incisions which only leave tiny scars – a good thing, of course. There is the same degree of prolonged swelling after surgery and there may be areas of permanent numbness over the cheeks and in the forehead. Movement of the face – particularly the eyebrows and occasionally the mouth – may be restricted afterwards, but this is usually temporary.

Like the ordinary mask lift, the endoscopic lift produces a radical change in the shape of your face. It is no good for jowls or for the neck region, so it is most often performed on younger patients unhappy with the upper two-thirds of their face.

Preparing for a face-lift

You can do a lot to maximise the potential of a face-lift. Lose weight, if you need to, before surgery, and then try to avoid a yo-yo pattern of weight gain and loss, which shows up in lax facial skin. Smoking impairs the circulation and robs the body of vitamin C, both of which are important for healing.

So stop smoking altogether if you can, or cut down two to three weeks before surgery and stop a week before the operation. Take a gram of vitamin C twice daily for at least two weeks beforehand, as well.

Alcohol makes bruising worse, so cut right down on drink. Bruising may be reduced by arnica, so it's worth taking one tablet four times a day for a week beforehand. Aspirin interferes with blood clotting, so don't take any for two weeks prior to the operation and for three weeks afterwards. (Many proprietary painkillers and flu remedies contain aspirin.)

If you are having surgery in the morning you should have nothing to eat or drink from midnight and do not put cream or make-up on your face in the morning.

The after effects

After surgery, you may have tight bandages and drains which will be removed the following day. Immediate complications include the development of swellings where blood accumulates and clots under the skin (haematoma). These must be drained or removed under anaesthesia.

Stitches are removed in five to 12 days. Your face will feel bruised, swollen, tight, numb and stiff for at least 14 disappointing and painful days and you may suffer from headaches and itching. You will be able to wash your hair within days of surgery.

You may also feel depressed. You may feel miserable simply because you look so awful. You may be anxious about the swelling – in case it's abnormal. You may feel guilty about having spent so much money pampering to your vanity. Or you may be simply unlucky and suffer frustrating complications which slow down healing so you can't get on with your life.

Witchhazel compresses help reduce swelling and it is best to sleep supported by several pillows so your head and chest are upright for a few days. Try to keep your head and neck as still as possible. In particular, try to avoid bending the neck forwards. Extra virgin olive oil, which is rich in vitamin E, may be used as a cold compress to speed the healing process. Sedatives and painkillers may be prescribed if necessary. And ultrasound is sometimes used, because the high energy vibrations seem to help prevent scarring, particularly under the neck.

You can wear make-up once stitches in front of the ears have been removed on the fifth day after surgery. Larger sutures in the scalp are taken out on the twelfth day and by two weeks bruising on the face and eyes has usually improved, so you can start to face the world again, though you may still feel tired.

Most people are back at work three weeks after surgery and you'll look fine in around two months. But during this time, your face will feel tight and you will be advised to avoid sport, any other strenuous activity or prolonged exposure to the sun. It's important to keep skin well moisturised. The full benefits may take another three months (six months for the mask lift) to show up.

Numbness of the cheeks, neck and around the ears from damage to nerve endings usually wears off in around three months when the sensory nerve grows back into the skin again. Any injury to the motor nerves connected with the movement of the mouth and eyebrows takes six weeks' recovery and is unlikely to be permanent.

The risks

Very rarely, a patient may be left with enduring pain in the cheeks or ears, numbness, or a lopsided smile due to weakness or even paralysis of part of one side of the face.

Additional side effects of a face-lift include changes in the colour of the skin – a darkening over sites of bruising, the development of red spider veins and a change of hair pattern. Moving the skin of the face alters the hairline so men sometimes find they have to shave behind their ears. Hair loss can also occur in the scalp near any incisions. It usually regrows after three months but not always. Occasionally the earlobes are distorted.

Scars are mostly hidden behind and in front of the ear, where there is a natural crease, in the hair and under the jaw, if work was done on the neck. All scars look red and angry at first. But they usually fade, unless wounds were stretched or became infected. Healing is often slowest of all under the chin.

Some people simply don't heal well and scars may become inflamed, itchy, thickened and lumpy (this includes lumps in the cheeks). People's healing abilities cannot be predicted but smokers and black people are much more likely to be left with bad scarring after surgery.

A form of gangrene (necrosis), which most commonly occurs behind the ear, is a very rare complication affecting skin which has lost its blood supply. This can cause bad scarring requiring further surgery.

It's hardly surprising that many people who have just had a face-lift feel miserable at first. After an operation to improve their appearance they first have to cope with looking worse than ever before for several days. But after the face settles down, when most people are beginning to appreciate how much better they look, some people remain disappointed.

They may have put themselves into the hands of an unskilled surgeon who has destroyed the symmetry of their appearance. Or they may have had unrealistic expectations of what surgery could do. A face-lift will not give you a different face if you're unhappy with the one you've got. Nor will it restore the health and vitality of your youth. A face-lift does not stop the clock. Lines, wrinkles and sagging will continue to develop and some people choose to have another face-lift further down the line.

After a face-lift you will look younger. You will then go on ageing and after some years you will be back to where you were – but, of course, you will be older. Thus, after one face-lift you will always look better than if you had never had one at all.

DEFINING THE JAWLINE

DOUBLE CHIN

Removing fat with liposuction (*see page 138*) is often enough to restore a sharp jawline to a younger person who has developed a double chin. This is done by inserting a fine tube into very small incisions hidden in the crease beneath the chin or behind each ear and sucking out the fat. A helmet of elasticated bandage must then be worn for two to three weeks to compress skin into shape. However, liposuction only works well for people with good skin tone, where skin will spring back after fat is sucked out.

Liposuction is not able to reach the fat which is deposited on the deeper side of the platysma muscle in the neck and it can leave the area feeling numb. There is also a risk of damaging the nerve that works the lips, leaving you with a lopsided smile. Additionally, most older people who have padding removed from this area will be left with jowls and a turkey gobble neck which look looser and worse than before.

TURKEY GOBBLE NECK

Older people with the loose skin that creates a turkey gobble neck – two vertical bands of excess skin – will need to have the excess skin removed as part of a face-lift. The cut is concealed beneath the chin. At the same time, the surgeon can also reach the underlying muscle – the fan-shaped platysma muscle – to tighten it and then cut it to restore a sharp right angle to the jaw.

Recovery from surgery to the neck takes around three to six months. It can cause a lot of bruising and a feeling of constriction around the neck. In addition, scars beneath the jaw take a particularly long time to soften and mature. They may be quite noticeable and feel stiff and lumpy for many weeks.

BUILDING UP THE CHIN

Creating a clean right angle between chin and neck is sometimes made easier by having your chin augmented. A weak or receding chin can be the reason for developing a double chin in the first place. Chin augmentation is often done in combination with surgery on the nose (*see page 40*) to balance the profile.

You can even ask for a cleft or dimple to be added and a large chin can also sometimes be modified by the removal of or altering of the bone.

Chin implants are usually made of silicone and can be inserted either from under the chin or through the mouth so there's no visible scar. But Gore-Tex, the membrane used to make hiking clothes weatherproof (*see page 87*), is also being used as a soft implant. However, implants can get infected, they can slip out of position and they can damage the sensation of the lower lip.

In addition, a chin implant puts pressure on the bone itself, sometimes causing the bone to dissolve so it recedes more than it did in the first place. In such cases, the implant can be removed and the jaw bone advanced.

This is a much more complicated procedure in which the surgeon makes a horizontal slice through the jaw bone and brings forward the bottom section.

HORIZONTAL NECK LINES

Nothing much can be done surgically for the horizontal neck lines, like tree rings, which are there from birth, but cutting the platysma muscle will often soften the look of rings and a light peel may also help.

The neck, throat and upper chest region is extremely delicate and difficult to treat satisfactorily with dermabrasion and deep peeling (*see page 74*), which are, in general, too harsh for this area of skin. Light peeling (*see page 81*) may be helpful, but once you stop weekly treatments, skin will eventually revert to its original condition. Regular exfoliation or the use of Retin A cream *(see page 96)* may also be helpful, but in lower doses than on the face.

Cost: £3,000 to £10,000 for a complete facial overhaul including the eyes and brow

Risks: numbness (usually resolves in three to six months); visible scars (poor healing can be a problem); a look you're not happy with; nerve damage (rare)

Ideal age: 40-plus

Length of stay in hospital: one night minimum, two to three nights maximum

Anaesthetic: general or, rarely, a local with intravenous sedation

Other drugs: painkillers, sedatives, antibiotics if necessary, steroids if necessary

Discomfort levels: very high for three weeks

Time before the signs of surgery disappear: three months (SMAS), six months (mask)

Length of time results last: around ten years, though effects are semi-permanent

CHAPTER THREE

Resculpturing the Nose

If you're troubled by an ugly nose, then an operation to correct it (rhinoplasty) will transform your face. But it's no good having a fixed idea about shape and size as drastic change is not usually advisable.

You simply can't refine a bulbous nose right down to a chiselled one. If you think of noses like feet, then you can only go down or up (with the insertion of extra cartilage or a silicone implant) a size or two, although humps, tips and nostrils can all be adjusted.

The nose rarely causes any distress until adolescence, because it doesn't start to grow until the age of 13 or 14. So there's no point in having surgery until it has stopped growing at around 18 or 19 at the earliest, or a repeat operation may be necessary. Girls tend to stop growing at a younger age than boys, so they may be able to have nose surgery earlier, perhaps at 16 or so. However, early surgery is rare.

Adolescence is a time of enormous concern about appearance and many young people are insecure about relatively minor problems of body image. They usually need reassurance rather than surgery, which should be strictly limited at this age to extreme cases only.

Improvement is nearly always possible, but perfection is not, so people who go along to a cosmetic surgeon clutching a photograph of their ideal nose will be disappointed. There is no such thing as an ideal, perfect, beautiful or even normal nose. The nose is part of your face and if it is in harmony with the rest of your features, then it will never be noticed.

Nose refinement is one of the most common cosmetic operations of all. If you think of the nose like a tent, then you can alter the shape of it by removing, changing or adding to the underlying structure of bone and cartilage (like tent poles) and redraping the skin over it.

The upper one-third of the nose consists of a pyramid of bone and the lower two-thirds consists of cartilage. The lower third of this cartilage consists of two domes which together create the shape of the all-important tip of the nose (*see the diagram below*).

No one has a nose that is completely straight or symmetrical. Many people have a twist in their septum – the partition inside the nose that divides it into two chambers.

The nose is our front line of defence against pollution and disease. It's our organ of smell and it moistens the air we breathe. Any damage to it may alter the airway and cause irritation giving us a runny or blocked up nose, when the lining swells up.

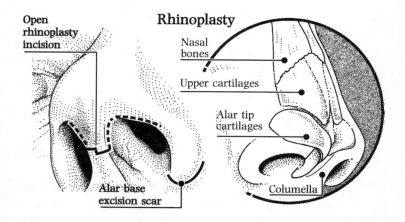

Open rhinoplasty incision

Rhinoplasty

Nasal bones

Upper cartilages

Alar tip cartilages

Columella

Alar base excision scar

The nose is sometimes injured at birth during difficult deliveries. When we are older, it may be damaged in an accident. And people who sniff a lot of cocaine may damage the inside of their nose so it collapses.

People who want surgery on their nose may want to repair an injured nose. They may want to modify the appearance of an ugly or distinctly ethnic nose. Or they may want secondary surgery to improve on poor results from an earlier operation. Some people may want to rejuvenate their nose.

As we age, there may be a drooping of the tip of the nose because the fat in the area has been partially absorbed and because skin has thinned, so the cartilage at the tip bulges out more. When this happens, the tip can be tilted up slightly to create a more youthful appearance.

PREPARING FOR NOSE SURGERY

After deciding that you want to change your nose, you must tell your surgeon (*see page 201*) at your first consultation exactly what it is that you want to alter – it's no good simply saying that you don't like your nose and want a better or a different one.

The type of nose that suits you will depend on the shape and length of your face, particularly the jaw, and even your body shape. Somebody else's nose may look good in a photograph – but it looks good on that particular person in that particular context.

The surgeon should look at your nose, examining its physical features from both outside and in, using a torch and speculum, and then tell you how it might be changed for the better. This discussion is very important because what you want may be different from what the surgeon thinks is best – and this is partly technical, partly aesthetic.

You should be told about how the operation will be done, the recovery time and possible complications. Photographs should then be taken ready for the second consultation. You should never decide to have surgery on your nose without using these photos in the discussions about what is going to be done.

Some surgeons use a polaroid camera but the resulting photos do not produce enough detail or a true enough image for proper discussion. Lifesize photos can be extremely useful and there are surgeons who use computerised images to give you an idea of the kind of nose you will end up with after surgery, however these pictures can be misleading. Most important, never trust a surgeon who says to you, 'This is the nose I will give you.'

It's impossible to predict precisely how a nose reshaping operation will turn out – it depends partly on the thickness of the skin of your nose, for instance. Thicker skin is harder to redrape. Above all, it's a delicate procedure – a millimetre here and there makes all the difference to the end result.

The second consultation is vital because you do not want to be committed to surgery unless you are sure that you and the surgeon are in agreement about the aim of the operation. It should also be made clear to you that this aim may not necessarily be achieved.

What is involved

There are three types of surgery:

Rhinoplasty. A straightforward closed operation which is

carried out from inside the nose, so there is no visible external scar at all. This operation can be done whenever there isn't a problem with the tip of the nose.

External rhinoplasty. A bigger operation, which involves opening the nose out via a cut in the columella – the strip of tissue separating the nostrils. This results in a small scar that no one ever sees, unless you're looking up at the sky, and it is an area where scars heal and fade away very successfully. When the nose is to be narrowed or nostrils made smaller, there will be also tiny scars hidden in the creases where the nostrils join the cheek.

Tip surgery. When a full rhinoplasty is not required, this operation is done. Sometimes the chin needs to be altered as well (*see page 36*), to balance the profile.

Bone is easy for the surgeon to work with because it can be removed, broken and moved around. But cartilage is a delicate, springy substance which has a memory – that is, if the surgeon tries to push it around it tends to return to its original position.

Because the nose is a pyramid in shape, if it is simply planed down it will always end up much wider at the top. So what the surgeon does to retain its original narrowness is to break the nose and then push both sides in. This break can either be done from inside or by inserting a little chisel through tiny nicks in the skin between the eyes, and on the cheeks. These nicks heal up without leaving scars and do not require stitches.

How the nose tip is dealt with is crucial. The mark of a balanced nose is a tip that's in proportion. If too much of the cartilage is removed, the nose will look unnatural.

To reduce a large nose, the surgeon can't simply remove a

lot of cartilage, because it serves an important function, acting as a valve to keep it open for breathing. This is why you can't have a large nose turned into a small one.

In fact, for most nose reductions, the only way to achieve a really symmetrical nose is to adjust the tip first of all and then cut the bone down to suit the tip, which is what the best surgeons would do.

Sometimes it's not a case of reducing the amount that the nose sticks out, but a case of bringing the bases closer together, or even of adding height to a flattened nose. This can be done either by using cartilage, taken from the ear or a rib, or bone, usually taken from the skull just above the ear.

Alternatively, an artificial substance, such as solid silicone or Gore-Tex, may be used but the problem with these is that they tend to become infected and can ulcerate out of the skin. However, surgeons really prefer to work with the patient's own tissues, which will continue to survive as a living graft.

A secondary rhinoplasty to correct an earlier operation is more complicated and unpredictable because it often involves putting something back rather than taking it away. The operation is made more difficult because not only has the normal anatomy been disturbed by the first operation, but also the surgeon has to work through a lot of scar tissue inside the nose, making results less predictable.

The rhinoplasty itself takes one to two hours and is carried out under a general anaesthetic, usually with one night's stay in hospital. To reduce bleeding, your blood pressure will be brought down or you will be injected with adrenaline and your nose will be packed with cocaine. The operation is then carried out according to the surgeon's specific plan.

The surgeon may have to perform one of two procedures before beginning work on shaping your nose – an SMR (submucosal resection of the septum) or an SMD (submucosal diathermy of the turbinate bones) – which are done to keep airways clear. Any polyps (benign growths) found in the nose must also be removed.

The after effects

When you wake up you will find plaster of Paris or a plastic splint taped over your nose to hold the fractured bones in place. You will be sat up against pillows and given ice packs to help reduce the swelling around your eyes. (Bruising around your eyes is more marked if you smoke, so you are advised to stop before having the operation – *see Preparing for a face-lift on page 32*.)

There is surprisingly little discomfort after surgery. Packs of paraffin gauze inside the nose are used less frequently and will be removed the morning after the operation. Then you can go home.

Try to avoid sneezing, blowing the nose, very hot baths and hot food and drink. Do not attempt to clean inside the nose with cotton buds and, above all, do not peep under the plaster to see your new nose, which will be disappointingly swollen and distorted for a little while yet.

Any external stitches in the columella will be taken out in four days and the plaster will be removed in about ten days, after which you can go back to work, with the help of some camouflage make-up to hide residual bruises.

Your nose will feel numb and stiff and it will probably still be swollen. You may have to breathe through your mouth. It takes several months for all the swelling to go down, during which time you must protect your nose from sun and heat. Numbness of the tip may take six months to wear off.

Most people are delighted with their new nose, which will not achieve its finished look for around six months. So be patient before jumping to the conclusion that you've wasted your money.

Younger patients are often pleased with a radical transformation, although older patients generally prefer a more discreet change. A successful operation may achieve such a subtle alteration that no one ever remarks on your new nose, which should be taken as a compliment. What often happens is that other people do notice a change somewhere in your face but they can't quite put their finger on it, so you may often be asked whether you've changed your hairstyle or told how well you're looking.

'People used to be able to stare right up my nose,' says Sophie Roberts, a painter, who's 39. 'I'm tall and my nose was long with gaping nostrils. I'd always hated it since I was a teenager and was called Big Nose at school. I grew my hair long and never wore it off my face. I looked like an Afghan hound and I used to avoid being seen in profile.

> 'I dreamt of having it done, but thought cosmetic surgery was for film stars – until the day I asked my husband what he'd like best in the world. When he asked me the same question back, I told him I'd like my nose done. He couldn't believe it bothered me so much.
>
> 'The surgeon's opinion was that my nostrils were the problem, rather than the length of my nose, though he said it was also slightly twisted. He also said that he would not make a drastic change, just improve it so it blended in with my face.

'The operation was excellent, although I looked dreadful after it, with two black eyes. But a fortnight later, when the time came to have the plaster off, I was incredibly apprehensive. When it was removed, I couldn't believe the joy I felt when I looked at myself in the mirror, from all angles, including my profile. I was ecstatic and when I walked out I immediately got a wolf whistle.

'My nose was good right from the start, even though I was told it would take six months to be at its best. The nostrils are much smaller and more closed and my nose sticks out less and is very slightly shorter. It was a bit runny at first and felt a little numb but now, nine months on, all I can feel is a slight hardness beneath the tip when I touch it.

'I feel so much more confident about myself. My husband loves my new nose and my mother, who has exactly the same nose, was really happy for me. She would have loved to have hers done, too. The funny thing is, not one other person has noticed the change.'

The risks

As the swelling goes down and the shape of your nose changes subtly, you may decide that it's not perfect. Or you may not like it.

Every cosmetic surgeon produces the occasional nose which the patient does not like or is technically imperfect. Around one in 20 people who have a rhinoplasty may require touch-up surgery.

This can usually be done under a local anaesthetic as a day case – it's often just a case of shaving off a little more bone. However, it cannot be done for a whole year after the original operation. The nose must not be touched until scars have completely matured and softened.

Other complications are unusual. The most common is swelling around the nose which eventually settles down and can be helped by massage. Nose bleeds after surgery are rare, but they can happen and then the nose will need further packing. Infection is also rare but can occur, usually high up in the nose, for which antibiotics are required. Sometimes the nose is constantly runny after surgery – a condition called reactive rhinitis – but this should settle down within three to six months.

Much more common is the development of tiny broken capillaries where the skin has become thinner, so that, from a distance, the nose looks pinker. These spider veins can be treated (*see page 99*) at a later date. People with fairly dark skins may notice that the skin below their eyes becomes darker after a rhinoplasty. This can be dealt with later on with laser treatment(*see page 89*). Very occasionally the nose ends up more twisted after surgery.

'I had a riding accident when I was 15 and it left my nose banana-shaped, with a bump on the bridge and a twist to one side,' says Valerie Peterson, a physiotherapist who's 31. 'I had my jaw fixed at the time, but not my nose because my father thought that to leave it was character-forming. I also believed that I should come to terms with it but it always made me shy around men and I never felt very attractive. I used to try and do my hair so as to detract attention from my ugly nose.

'Around my thirtieth birthday, I decided to do something about it. My surgeon told me afterwards that it had taken him several attempts to break it with a mallet and chisel.

Then he reset it and I woke up with a plaster across the nose and a bib below it to catch the blood. It did not feel painful but my eyes were incredibly irritated, sore and uncomfortable and they swelled up like balloons. I looked monstrous. I went back a few days later to have the pads taken out of my nose, which meant that I could finally breathe through it again.

'Two weeks later, when the mask came off, I still had yellow bruising round my eyes and was still a little swollen, though make-up would have concealed it and I suppose I could have gone back to work.

'Anyway, I wasn't satisfied with what the operation had achieved – I still had a noticeable bump. So a year later, I had it operated on again, when the surgeon used a new modelling technique to open up the nose completely and reshape it.

'This time, of course, I was better prepared for the swelling and bruising and now I have a completely straight – well, not dead straight – nose. I need to use make-up on it to conceal the broken blood vessels caused by the surgery, but I'll get those fixed eventually.

'I do feel guilty about spending so much money on my nose – I paid £3,500 in all. But it's made such a difference to my life. My new nose makes me feel more confident. On a bad day I know I look normal and on a good day I feel really dashing.'

Cost: around £3,000

Risks: poor result, either because you dislike the new shape or because of bad surgery; a temporarily runny nose; and – though extremely rare – a breathing obstruction, which can be permanent

Length of stay in hospital: one night

Anaesthetic: general

Other drugs: none

Discomfort levels: low

Time before the signs of surgery disappear: three weeks

Length of time results last: permanent

CHAPTER FOUR

Eyes, Lips and Ears

RAISING THE EYEBROWS

There are two groups of muscle in the forehead – one which lifts the brow and one which pulls it down. The position of our eyebrows is determined by a balance between how we use these muscles (facial behaviour) and the force of gravity.

As muscles get weaker with age, our eyebrows gradually start to droop, causing excess skin to collect in the upper eyelids. And, because our skin gets thinner with age, facial muscles tend to become more visible through it – particularly the ones used for frowning at the top of the nose and those that create crow's feet. As a result, over the years, a severe, sad or tired expression, with a deep furrow between the eyebrows, often develops.

Many older women try to disguise drooping eyebrows by plucking them and others also consciously try to keep their eyebrows lifted up away from their eyes. This muscular action only adds to the development of horizontal lines across the forehead.

A heavy drooping brow can be raised with a brow-lift which entails cutting the muscle responsible for pulling it down. After a brow-lift operation, many women will say something along the lines of, 'I never realised how heavy my lids were until I had surgery.'

The operation does not, in general, act on the horizontal lines caused by raising the eyebrows nor will it totally erase the frown furrow, but a brow-lift will modify them and they can be treated separately with chemical peeling later (*see page 78*).

THE BROW-LIFT OPERATION

The surgeon used to cut an Alice band incision from ear to ear. This open brow procedure has a high complication rate, frequently causing hair loss across the broad scar. Nerves which supply sensation are often cut, leaving numbness or an unpleasant feeling of ants crawling across the scalp.

Today, the operation may be carried out endoscopically – a tiny camera and lights are passed through small incisions behind the hair under the skin and the operation is monitored on a TV screen. The skin is lifted off the bone and pulled up and the eyebrows gently restored to their original arch.

The muscle close to the nose that pulls the brow down is weakened and the tip of the nose is sometimes lifted at the same time to correct the droop that often occurs with ageing.

Pulling up the arch of the eyebrows has an immediate effect on excess skin overhanging the eye. Eyebrows are fixed in place either with surgical glue or screws (which are removed four to six days later). The surgeon should take great care to preserve the natural balance of the face and avoid creating a look of surprise.

Although the brow-lift is carried out under a general anaesthetic, a night in hospital is not required unless it is combined with a face-lift. Additional surgery – a face-lift and/or eyelid surgery – is often carried out at the same time as a brow-lift, and the pre- and post-operative care and many of the possible complications of a brow-lift are the same as for a face-lift (*see page 32*).

The risks

There is likely to be noticeable bruising which tends to run down from the eye area and show up most of all in the cheeks. The forehead will feel numb and there may be some tingling. There will also be very limited movement of the forehead. Normal sensation and the ability to raise your eyebrows will return in a week or so and hair will regrow around the incisions in three months.

The major risk of a brow-lift is damage to the natural movement of the forehead. If the forehead is totally smooth after the operation, then it means that the muscle which pulls the brow up has been paralysed. Another risk is being left with a lopsided look, where one eyebrow is noticeably lower than the other.

We are all lopsided to some extent and there is always more skin in one eyelid than the other, because that eyebrow is lower. Normally, we don't notice this at all. A brow-lift can usually iron out these tiny discrepancies. A common side effect of having the open operation is being left with abnormal sensation in the scalp.

The real problem for the surgeon is how to anchor brows so that their new position is retained. It's easy for the brow to droop back down again because the scalp is so mobile.

'I had a brow-lift done last June,' says Susanna Livingstone, a secretary who's 47. 'My boss first noticed that the skin over my right eye was drooping right down in a hood, then my son mentioned it and then I realised that when I looked up I could actually see the skin.

'I went to my GP and was referred to a hospital where I was told that the muscles had collapsed over my right eye and surgery would put it right. Well, I had the operation but a year or so later, the skin began to descend again. This time I was told that the only permanent way of fixing it was to have a brow-lift.

'I went in on Friday and was out on Sunday. I had the endoscopic operation – on the NHS – and I've been left with two gold pins in my head that can be taken out if I start getting headaches.

'My face was very swollen for a long time. I didn't go back to work for a month and even then I had to wear sunglasses to hide the bruising and swelling. After about two months I looked fine and so did my right eye, and that's when people started to say that I looked younger and less tired, which was a nice bonus, because I didn't have the operation for cosmetic purposes. So I am very pleased.'

Cost: £2,000 to £3,000

Risks: loss of ability to raise eyebrows; lopsidedness; a surprised look; baldness; pain in scalp

Ideal age: 35-plus

Length of stay in hospital: one night at most

Anaesthetic: IV sedation with local, or general

Other drugs: painkillers

Discomfort levels: medium

Time before the signs of surgery disappear: three months

Length of time results last: semi-permanent

BRIGHTENING UP THE EYES

Men and women who have hoods, bags or fatty pouches around the eyes often have to suffer other people's comments about how tired they look or suggestions that they must have been out on the town the night before. Anyone who works in entertainment or the media will also be aware of just how noticeable these hoods, bags and pouches are under intense lighting.

Having the excess skin and fat cut away from above and below the eyelids can instantly make women and men – who are particularly prone to surplus skin around the eyes – look more fresh-faced and wide awake. And it can sometimes be achieved without anyone ever guessing that they've had cosmetic surgery, because the operation can occasionally be done from the inside of the lower eyelids, so there are no visible scars.

The operation is called blepharoplasty and it can brighten you up on its own but it is often carried out at the same time as a brow-lift and/or a face-lift which, done together, will create a harmonious look, will mean one episode of swelling and bruising and will make everything cheaper. Blepharoblasty can also be carried out to add a crease to the upper lids of Oriental people, who desire a more Western look.

What to expect

Eyelid surgery will remove bags and excess skin but will not eradicate creases, such as crow's feet, though the lines will be softened, especially if the surgeon tightens the muscle that creates them at the same time. It is normal for the face to crease when you smile and laugh.

Neither will the operation improve cheek bags, which are sometimes actually made worse by eyelid surgery, especially if you smoke. Dark circles under the eyes can be lightened by laser treatment (*see page 90*) or chemical peeling (*see page 78*) in a separate procedure.

You rarely have to stay overnight in hospital since the operation is carried out either under sedation and a local anaesthetic or as a day case under general anaesthetic.

The eye is our organ of vision. It is a ball which sits in a bony socket, cushioned by fat, supported by ligaments and moved by muscles. There is a film of tear fluid across the front of our eyes, which is changed all the time by our eyelids, which act a little like windscreen wipers.

Tears are produced in a gland in the top of the upper eyelid and drained away through the tear duct in the inner corner of the lower lid. There is also a small tear duct in the upper lid.

The eyelid itself consists of skin lined with mucous membrane. It has its own layer of fat and its own set of muscles which open and close it. As we age, the ligaments supporting the fat in the eyelid weaken. This causes the fat to drop down and settle into a bag where the skin is thin. The surgeon will not be working on the actual eyeball, but the operation can affect the tear film.

Many people decide to have their eyelids done at a time when they are starting to wear glasses for long sight. If you are considering eyelid surgery, then you're advised to get your vision checked first, even though what the surgeon does will not affect the function of your eyes.

It's also important to bring any medical problems affecting your eyes to the attention of your surgeon – for example, whether they are dry or excessively watery, or you've worn contact lenses for a long time. Other problems include having had glaucoma, a detached retina, surgery for a squint, or a weak, drooping upper lid (ptosis) or thyroid problems which affect the eyes.

TIGHTENING UP THE TOP LIDS

The usual problem is one of too much skin. This may be caused by drooping brows – for which a brow-lift (*see page 52*) is more effective than eyelid surgery – but the surgeon should also check for a drooping lid, which requires a different operation. When you gaze straight ahead, the upper lid should rest at the level of the top of the iris, not at the level of the pupil.

The surgeon cuts – with extreme care – a long ellipse of skin from along the line of the upper eyelid crease. Where there is hooding on the outer side of the eye (which may also be helped by a brow-lift) the cut will extend further out into the crow's feet. Along with the skin, the surgeon also removes fat which accumulates beneath the muscle responsible for screwing up the eye.

The operation leaves a long thin scar which rarely causes problems other than little lumps (cysts) which soon clear up. It's difficult for a surgeon to go wrong with this procedure, although there is a small risk of damage to the muscle opening the eye, leading to a drooping lid, and an even smaller risk of damage to the tear-film, resulting in a dry, gritty, reddened eye.

There is a danger of too much skin being taken out, making the eyelid too tight to close easily, and the operation is not always entirely successful in removing all of the fat on

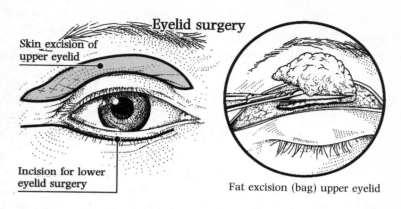

Eyelid surgery

Skin excision of upper eyelid

Incision for lower eyelid surgery

Fat excision (bag) upper eyelid

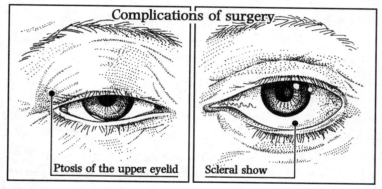

Complications of surgery

Ptosis of the upper eyelid | Scleral show

the inner side of the eye and all the hooding on the outer side.

Sometimes the lid continues to feel numb after surgery and feeling may not return for up to six weeks, but this numbness does not interfere with its movement.

GETTING RID OF THOSE BAGS

The usual problem with the lower lid is a weakness in the wall supporting the fat that pads out the eye, which leads to the development of fatty bags under the eyes. This weakness tends to develop with age, but sometimes it runs in families so that much younger people can have them.

Hence there are two types of operation: one for the young, who only need the fat removed, and the other for older people, who need excess skin removed as well as the fat.

When the surgeon is only removing fat, it is possible to do the operation from inside the lid, which means there will be no scars. An incision is made – sometimes with a laser – and the fat is teased out. If loose skin is also to be removed, then the operation must be done from outside. This is one of the hardest operations for the cosmetic surgeon to judge. A cut is made immediately below the lashline (where eyeliner is applied) and out into the crow's feet and then the decision must be made on how much the lid needs to be tightened and how much fat must be removed.

Too tight – and the lid may come away from the eye, causing it to dry out. Or it might reveal too much white of the eye (scleral show) or cause eyes to become rounder than before. Removing too much fat can cause 'empty' eye sockets, which will make you look as if you're starving.

The newest technique is not to take all the fat out, but to redrape it in the groove beneath the eye. The swelling after the operation lasts longer when this is done, but it leaves a more natural look.

The after effects of eye surgery

Following eye surgery, there will be swelling and bruising around the eyes, which usually subsides within about ten days, with the help of ice packs and compresses of witchhazel or extra virgin olive oil. Stitches are removed three to five days later and scars must be protected from strong sunlight for several months.

Eyes will water a lot and they will feel gritty, tight, itchy and swollen. There will also be a loss of sensation in the lids (women who apply eye make-up will notice this) until the nerves grow back into the skin, which takes around twelve weeks.

The risks

Sometimes fluid accumulates beneath the mucous membrane covering the front of the eye after surgery. This condition (subconjunctival oedema) makes the eye glisten and water and may last four to five weeks. If it's bad, the surgeon can snip the membrane to release the fluid.

Scars may become red and swell up, which could last for several months, though they can be disguised with make-up at the end of the first week and they will eventually fade right away. Little lumps may also develop in the scars, but they usually disappear on their own.

The contraction of the skin caused by scarring can also make it hard to shut the eyes completely. This causes eyes to dry out and become red and sore. Moist swabs over the eyes, taping them shut at night and the use of artificial tears (not commercial eye drops) can ease this condition, which should put itself right as the swelling goes down, but further surgery is occasionally required.

As mentioned, where too much skin is removed from the lower lids, you may be left showing a lot of white in the lower part of the eye. This is a particular risk for people who smoke or who have worn contact lenses for many years –

their lower eyelids have become weakened and so are unable to support the lid effectively.

An unskilled surgeon may accidentally damage the muscle that opens and closes the upper eyelids so that one droops. Some people complain that the shape of their eyes has changed after eyelid surgery or that their eyes have become slightly rounder as a result of the surrounding skin being pulled out instead of up.

But we all have slightly asymmetric eyes. None of us have exactly the same amount of skin and fat below each eye and a surgeon cannot guarantee that there will be absolutely no change in shape.

The subtle alteration which can occur to the shape of your eyes after a blepharoblasty is rarely noticeable to anyone other than yourself. If you feel very strongly that your eyes are your best feature and you don't want the appearance of them to alter in any way, then don't have a blepharoblasty.

The operation does not affect your vision, but it may have an effect on the film of tears covering the eyes and this can either improve your vision, or make it worse. People who have had a lot of excess skin removed from their top lids usually report that their vision is easier now the heaviness has gone. Blindness as a result of eyelid surgery is extremely rare.

'I had my eyes done eight years ago,' says Elizabeth Collins, who's now 60 and still working as an office manager. 'I always had bags under my eyes and slack skin which hung down over my eyes, and I really wanted to get rid of all that – and, my God, surgery made such a difference.

'The surgeon simply cut underneath my bottom lashes and in the lid line on top, but the marks were so fine I could hardly see them, even immediately after the operation. I remember I had to have some stitches – which were so tiny I could hardly see those either – removed four to five days later and my eyes were puffy and bruised for two weeks or so. But there are no scars whatsoever. And my eyes look the same now as they did when I was in my twenties.'

Cost: (upper lids under local): £1,000; (lower lids under local): £1,250; (both, under local anaesthetic): £2,000; (both, under general): £2,500

Risks: watering of the eyes; inability to close the eyes causing dry eyes; a subtle change of look; rounder eyes; more white of the eye showing

Ideal age: any age

Length of stay in hospital: none

Anaesthetic: local or as a day case under general anaesthetic

Other drugs: painkillers

Discomfort levels: high

Time before the signs of surgery disappear: three months

Length of time results last: semi-permanent

HOLLYWOOD LIPS

Narrowing and lengthening of the lips is a feature of the ageing face. Unfortunately there is no foolproof way to augment thin lips, which is what many younger women also want today, thanks to the fashion for the beestung mouth (Paris lip).

You shouldn't use silicone in lips, so most people opt for collagen injections (*see page 83*). These can be carried out both in the lips themselves and in the upper rim of the lip to define the cupid's bow. Here, the collagen runs along the outer line very satisfactorily, but since there is so much movement of the mouth, it is rapidly absorbed and really does not last long at all, making treatment expensive, as you have to go back for a top up every month or so. The edge of the lips can be further defined by permanent make-up (*see page 103*), although injections are painful in this area.

Fat is occasionally injected in much the same way, and often disappears. Silicone should not be injected into the lips because it hardens and is rejected. A permanent alternative is to pass a thread of Gore-Tex (*see page 87*) down the centre of each lip. The thread can be felt by the person who's had it done, but not by anyone who happens to kiss those lips.

The surgical alternatives

Surgically, the most common way of plumping out a thin upper lip is with a graft of fat. The top layer of skin (epidermis) is removed from the area where the fat is to come from – usually the abdomen or buttocks – and an ellipse of dermis, with some fat attached, is cut out. This is curled up and slid into a tunnel hollowed out of the upper lip.

This procedure leaves a scar at the place the graft was taken and the lip may occasionally become infected and the graft may not take and might need to be removed. However, if it is successful, it's the best way.

'I was a model working in Singapore, where big Hollywood lips are fashionable,' says Angie Hudson, who's 25. 'So I decided to have my top lip enhanced.

'I came back to England to have it done and the surgeon said he would take the fat graft from my belly, where I already have a scar from having my appendix out. He also said he could tidy up the old scar at the same time.

'He measured my lip, marked it out and injected it with local anaesthetic. Then he measured a strip of skin next to my appendix scar and cut it out. He made three small cuts inside my top lip – the next part was horrible as he tunnelled through the lip and I could feel him pulling inside. But then he put in some little stitches and said that was that.

'Well, my lip was incredibly swollen and bruised and tender for days. It was really annoying, being over here and unable to kiss my boyfriend. One of the stitches fell out almost immediately and the others fell out two weeks later, by which time my lip was more or less OK. But the problem was that it was now really big, especially in the middle, and I didn't like it at all.

'When I went back to the surgeon, he just said it would go down in time, but it didn't. So nine months later, I went to see another surgeon, who made an adjustment to my lip, trimming it down under local anaesthetic. This did reduce its size, but when the cut healed the scar was uneven – so now I've got an uneven top lip.

'Yet another surgeon has advised me to have a third operation to correct this unevenness but I am scared now that it will just make it worse. I wish I'd never had anything done to my lip in the first place.'

Lips may also be given a more pronounced pout by removing

a narrow strip of skin from the lip rim (where lip liner is applied), so that when the wound heals and contracts in a scar, the lips roll outwards. This procedure usually results in a noticeable scar that is hard to disguise with lipstick and may be asymmetrical, resulting in a crooked mouth.

Fleshy lips can be reduced by the reverse procedure – removing a strip of mucosa and fat from the inside of the lips so they roll inwards. This operation is occasionally sought by black people.

To help correct loose skin at the corners of an older person's mouth, an ellipse of skin is cut from the corner leaving a permanent scar that requires disguise with make-up. This procedure is not successful.

Cost: (dermal fat grafts, upper only): £750; (both lips) £1,250

Risks: poor result, loss of graft

Ideal age: any age

Length of stay in hospital: none

Anaesthetic: local (or day-case general)

Other drugs: mild painkillers

Discomfort levels: medium

Time before the signs of surgery disappear: two to six weeks

Length of time results last: variable

EAR-PINNING

Everyone's ears are completely different. They differ from other people's and they differ on each side. Ears are so unique that the authorities were originally thinking of using them for purposes of identity.

Ears that stick out attract attention. Children with noticeably prominent ears are often taunted at school, and are sometimes labelled as stupid. And the stigma attached to noticeable ears means that many parents feel they should book their children in early for an ear-pinning operation (otoplasty). Prominent ears tend to run in families and the parents may have suffered in their youth.

More deformed ears are often small and low down on the side of the head because ears develop in the embryo from tissue on the side of the neck and move up to the side of the head. One such congenital abnormality is where the ears are small and rather cup-like in shape.

Much more common are minor abnormalities where the ears stick out, or bat ears. In some cases, these have not formed what's called the antehelical fold. This is the fold in the cartilage that lies between the rim of the ear and the ear canal. It helps us decide the direction from which a sound is coming. In other cases, there is simply too much cartilage around the ear canal, pushing the ear out.

There is now a new technique of splinting abnormal ears in the first few days of life. When a baby is being born, the mother produces a hormone called relaxin which allows her pubic bone to widen and let the baby through. Babies absorb this hormone so that immediately after birth the cartilage in their ears is soft and malleable and can be moulded by wire and taped to the head to create a normal shape, thus avoiding the need for an operation later on.

However, many doctors are unaware of this procedure and it is rarely carried out at present. An ear-pinning operation should not be done before the age of four or five, because the cartilage has not yet stiffened. It is difficult to decide exactly when to operate because the ears often reach full size at about six or seven. However, it is worth remembering that at such a young age, however much surgery is intended to ensure the child's emotional wellbeing, it is the parents who decide to have it done, not the child. And in most cases, it should be left to the child to decide when he or she is old enough whether or not to have surgery.

What is involved

A younger child will have surgery as a day case under a general anaesthetic, but with adults and older children earpinning is usually done under local anaesthetic.

The aim of surgery will be either to create an antehelical fold, which bends back the top part of the ear, or, more frequently, to remove some of the excess cartilage which makes the whole ear stick out. Sometimes the surgeon will do both at once.

It is easy for people to lose a lot of blood from their ears so it is vital that no aspirin is taken for at least a fortnight prior to surgery. The ear is marked out and injected with adrenaline to stop bleeding and local anaesthetic. This means that although the patient does not feel the operation, he or she can hear what is going on extra loudly.

The surgeon will make a cut in the back of the ear and burrow through the cartilage under the front skin of the ear and make cuts in the cartilage which allow a fold to be created. Cartilage is springy stuff so it must be held in place with stitches. When there is too much cartilage an ellipse of it is removed from the base of the ear.

The back of the ear is stitched and a dressing of cotton

wool or sponge is applied to cushion and splint the ear to the head. For the first couple of days, the ears will feel very sore and the patient should rest at home so there is no risk of bleeding. The dressing must remain on for ten days, then it will be removed to have any non-dissolving stitches taken out. The ears will be flat but bruised and red. They should still be kept flat at night with a headband.

The risks

Sometimes the skin on the front of the antehelical fold breaks down but this usually heals up again of its own accord. Other complications include bleeding, the development of haematoma (collections of clotted blood under the skin) which might need removal, painful ears (during exertion or cold weather) and the development of thick, hard scar tissue (keloid scars).

Surgical over-correction or under-correction can leave ears completely flattened or with just the top or bottom sticking out. This can make them look worse than before.

Ear-pinning can be particularly important for men, because their ears are normally on show. It can also help women who want to wear their hair short, up or back off their face.

'My ears stuck out so much that I would never wear my hair up or back or have it short. I particularly hated my left ear, which stuck out more than the other one,' says 38-year-old Joanna Anderson, who's a plant breeder.

> 'I went to see a surgeon and he talked me out of having both my ears done. He said that making the left one match the right would be sufficient. I had it done under a local anaesthetic and felt no pain at all, even though I could hear the surgeon crunching and slicing.

'Afterwards I felt fine. My ear throbbed a bit and I couldn't press on it. But I had to wear this polystyrene dressing for two weeks, during which time I couldn't hear a thing on that side. Luckily I wasn't working at the time and could wear a hairband to cover the dressing. But it must be incredibly hard for children having both ears done at once.

'Two weeks later the dressing came off. The ear took a little while to settle down. It's still a bit numb, six months on. But it's great to have symmetrical ears. The surgeon was quite right, he didn't pin the left one flat to the head at all. They simply match and now they don't seem to stick out at all.'

Cost: around £1,000 for two ears, under local anaeshetic

Risks: bleeding; skin breakdown; painful ears; poor result

Ideal age: from five onwards

Length of stay in hospital: none

Anaesthetic: general (young children); local (adults)

Other drugs: mild painkillers

Discomfort levels: medium

Time before the signs of surgery disappear: three weeks

Length of time results last: permanent

EARLOBE SURGERY

Surgeons are often asked to remove the itchy, hard, lumpy (keloid) scars that can form after ear-piercing. Simply cutting out the lump is not the answer since another keloid scar will probably develop. So surgeons will either use superficial radiotherapy, injections of steroids or pressure to break up the scar tissue.

Occasionally, as part of the ageing process, people's ear-lobes become much longer and droopier – especially if they have been constantly weighed down by heavy earrings. So, as part of a face-lift or even on its own, the surgeon can remove a wedge from the earlobe – like cutting a slice out of a cake – and stitch up the small wound, which usually heals quickly and satisfactorily. This can be done under local anaesthesia.

CHAPTER FIVE

Alternatives to the Knife

IRONING OUT THE FOREHEAD

The latest technique to smooth a furrowed brow is to inject it with botulinum toxin, instead of having a brow-lift which involves surgery *(see page 53)*. Botulinum toxin is a chemical which causes a temporary paralysis of the muscles and has been used by doctors for some years to treat people with facial twitches.

It works by blocking a naturally occurring chemical which causes muscle fibres to contract and now cosmetic surgeons are using it to 'freeze' the upper part of the face in order to relax horizontal forehead lines, vertical frown lines and even crow's feet.

Four precisely placed injections are needed for horizontal forehead lines and two for vertical frown lines or crow's feet. Injecting the wrong muscle can cause the eyebrow to droop, for which nothing can be done until the effects of the botulin wear off.

Results are noticeable five days after the injections and last for three to six months. During this time muscles become smaller and less obvious because they are not being used and wrinkles relax away. Some people even learn to stop lifting their brow.

The lines may simply drop out or the dents can be filled in with collagen *(see page 83)*. However, once the botulin wears off, most people are back to square one and will need repeat injections.

'I was always screwing up my face,' says 41-year-old Sarah Ireland, who's a history teacher. 'My sister used to ask me why I was always frowning. In the end I started wearing a fringe to conceal the lines across and down my forehead.

'I first had a go with collagen injections but I noticed that afterwards it hurt when I frowned, so I stopped frowning for six weeks or so while the collagen lasted, which gave me the idea for having the botulin treatment.

'I had it done two months ago. All I felt was a few pricks where I was injected along the lines of my forehead and between my eyes. On the fifth day, I found I simply couldn't frown anymore, so the lines are much more shallow and have nearly disappeared.

'In three months' time or so I'll have some more injections and then again twice more, which will make four treatments altogether and I think by that time I will have completely forgotten how to frown.

'I highly recommend this treatment and when I told one of my friends about it, she went and had her crow's feet done. She looks fine now, not that the lines were that noticeable to start with.'

Cost: £150 plus consultation fee.

Risks: temporarily drooping eyebrow

Length of stay in hospital: none

Anaesthetic: none

Other drugs: none

Discomfort levels: none

Time before the signs of surgery disappear: no surgery so almost immediate improvement

Length of time results last: six months

DERMABRASION AND PEELING

These two treatments strip off the top layers of skin along with all the blemishes and superficial wrinkles. Dermabrasion can be compared with sandpapering or planing wood, peeling is more like using paintstripper. The aim is to expose new skin, which will heal into a smooth flat surface with some of the properties of youthful skin, such as no creases.

Both procedures remove the epidermis (the horny outer layer of skin) and part of the dermis below. This damage encourages the skin to reconstruct itself and promotes the production of collagen, the skin's scaffolding. Neither procedure has any effect on sagging skin nor on the nose-to-mouth grooves. Results depend on how deeply the skin has been penetrated.

The major drawback of dermabrasion and peeling is that they both cause enlarged pores and discolouration and bleaching in the treated area, leaving a tide mark at the edges. Discolouration and bleaching occur because the treatments damage the melanocytes – cells which produce the brown pigment (melanin) that gives skin its colour and makes it tan in the sun – which are found in the lowest layer of the epidermis. The deeper any treatment goes in the skin the more likely there is to be a complication.

DERMABRASION

A method of mechanically sanding away the top layer of skin, dermabrasion is used to try and remove many types of skin blemish including acne pits, scars and chickenpox scars, as well as brown patches and superficial fine lines. It penetrates most deeply and is best at treating creases in the skin, such as the pucker marks that develop around the lips, causing lipstick to 'bleed'.

Sometimes more than one treatment is required to smooth skin down to the level of deep acne pits, for example, or a chemical peel may be done at the same time to increase penetration.

'My acne started when I was ten and cleared up when I was 17, leaving me with severe scars on my forehead, in particular,' says Celia Mitchell, a town planner who is now 29.

'I always wore my hair in a thick fringe and I hated the wind blowing it off my face so my bumpy skin showed. When I was 20 I went to my GP because I was upset about my appearance.

'I was referred to a plastic surgeon who recommended dermabrasion. But the NHS waiting list is long and it took a year before I was told to come into hospital the following day. I felt so nervous and unsure about what I was letting myself in for that I didn't go, nor did I go the second time my name came up a year or two later.

'So in the end I went to see a surgeon privately at a time, six years ago, when I was between jobs, knowing I wouldn't have to worry about taking time off or people at work knowing what I'd had done.

'I had my forehead dermabraded, which I remember as being pretty painful but it was quite successful so I decided to have it done again.

'This time, six months ago, I had my whole face done except for my nose and chin area. The operation took 50 minutes. I had a general anaesthetic and when I woke up I felt fine, so I went home, my face covered in lint. Over the next few days I could feel the skin underneath itching, so I knew it was healing.

'On the seventh day, I soaked the lint off to reveal smooth, new, pink skin. At first it was so swollen that the skin was completely smooth. But over three weeks, as the swelling went down, I could see the residual scarring come back again.

'I'm still left with some scarring and I still won't wear my hair back off my face but now I don't mind when the wind blows my fringe back to reveal the skin. I do look rather pale, because my skin is slightly lighter and because I've been wearing sunblock.

'I paid over £1,000 for my face to be done. Of course I should have been braver and had it done on the NHS but I think the money was well-spent. I just should have had it done earlier.'

What is involved

Dermabrasion is carried out as a day case under local or general anaesthetic, depending on the extent of the area to be sanded. The instrument used is a small rotating wire brush or diamond wheel. There will be bleeding and skin will be painful and swollen for a week to ten days after the operation. A scab will develop after a couple of days and lift off in seven to ten days, depending on the depth of the sanding, after which make-up can be gently applied.

The newly exposed skin is highly delicate and an angry red to start with, but as it reconstructs itself and starts to mature, the pinkness will disappear over the course of three months or so.

During this time it is essential to protect the skin from the sun with sunblock and from any stress and strain caused by exertion, cold wind or infection. Scaling and itching can be eased with a mild moisturising cream.

The risks

Tiny whiteheads called milia sometimes develop three to four weeks after the operation. These can be removed with a rough flannel or they may just disappear. The skin will never tan properly again and must always be protected from the sun.

Dermabrasion is a form of extreme exfoliation and can achieve soft, smooth and slightly shiny-looking skin. But it is often pale and blotchy in colour. And the treatment must be carried out by an experienced surgeon with a steady hand who knows exactly how deep to penetrate. Sanding too deep can cause permanent and very obvious scars.

'I first noticed the pucker marks on my upper lip about seven or eight years ago,' says Elizabeth Collins, an office manager who's now 60, 'and they continued to get worse as my lip shrank, turning into real ridges – like corrugated iron. I kept rubbing in cream and taking cod liver oil but they did no good at all. I smoke three cigarettes a day and have done so since I was 20, so that may have had something to do with it.

'I had my upper lip dermabraded last year. It was done at the same time as a face-lift, so I had a general anaesthetic. When I woke up, my lip felt mildly sore and it looked just like a knee looks when you've grazed it badly. There was a pinky red smooth line along the top of my lip. A few little scabs developed, which fell off within a week and that was that. Not a mark, nor a scar remained. The skin was the same colour as the rest of my face. I had a perfect upper lip once more.'

CHEMICAL PEELS

The outcome of a peel also depends on the degree of penetration. The deeper a surgeon goes, the more likely complications will develop. The deepest peel is achieved using the corrosive chemical phenol, which is toxic and can affect the heart and kidneys and will cause burns if it goes too deep. The other chemical used is trichloroacetic acid (TCA), which is more predictable and comes in different strengths.

Preparation of the skin is very important. Before a peel, skin must be primed for four weeks with daily applications of strong Retin A cream (*see page 96*). You may be advised to apply a solution of bleach daily, as well, to try and shut down the melanocytes and protect them from damage.

Results also depend partly on your skin type. Fair-skinned people and thin-skinned people do best.

What is involved

Phenol is not used much today, but when it is the patient must be sedated. After application, the face is pressure-bandaged with white elastoplast for 48 hours. When the tape is removed, the outer layer of skin comes off with it – causing excruciating pain.

A TCA peel does not require sedation, just the application of an anaesthetic cream 45 minutes beforehand, so it can be done as an outpatient. The skin has its natural grease removed with alcohol and then the acid is painted on. An electric fan helps relieve the pain. When the TCA has frosted, the peel is stopped. Iced saline, which takes the pain away, is run over the skin and then petroleum jelly is smeared all over.

Two days later, the skin is washed to decrease scabbing, which can promote infection and scarring. If a scar persists steroid cream or injections may be required to damp down redness and itching and prevent scarring.

As an anti-ageing procedure or for the removal of blemishes, a peel can work. But it does require commitment. You will not want anyone to see you for a few days and it may take up to three months before the redness completely disappears.

The risks

A peel has all the same drawbacks as dermabrasion. It can cause skin thinning, enlarged pores, permanent sun-sensitivity, discolouration and a bleached out complexion.

This new paleness may, on the positive side, get rid of dark shadows beneath the eyes but it may also commit you to wearing tinted make-up in public for the rest of your life. A peel also creates a visible tidemark, so you will need to blend in treated skin with make-up. As with dermabrasion, little whiteheads sometimes appear in the skin afterwards.

It is vital that a chemical peel is carried out by an expert who can assess the precise degree of penetration. Too deep a peel will mean permanent skin damage.

'I've had dermabrasion and two peels on an extremely deep line that developed in my upper lip after I had root canal treatment,' says Sandra Nielson, a novelist aged 62.

> 'The line was so deep that my lipstick would run right up to my nose. On one occasion a shop assistant asked me if I knew I had lipstick under my nose. So when my husband asked me what I wanted for my birthday, I said I wanted to get rid of the line.
>
> 'I found that both treatments, which covered a circular area from the base of my nose to my chin, caused terrible pain. After the dermabrasion my skin was bright red and I looked like a teddy bear. But it healed up very quickly and after 14 days you'd never know I'd had anything done.
>
> 'The second peel healed up after just ten days, even though the surgeon had put extra acid on the line which made it stand out red on my face. It's much better than it used to be, but you can still see traces of the line and I'm going back in six weeks to see if the surgeon can do another peel to get rid of it completely.'

If you decide to undergo dermabrasion or a chemical peel, you should stop taking the contraceptive pill for at least a month before treatment and a month afterwards to reduce the risk of discolouration in the treated areas.

If you're a vegetarian, be warned. Your diet may impair your ability to heal normally. US surgeons at a meeting of the American Academy of Cosmetic Surgery recently described two cases of vegetarians who experienced delayed healing or unexpected scarring after chemical peels. This is thought to be due to a nutritional imbalance causing lowered production of a substance called hydroxyproline, which is essential for healing wounds.

Cost (for localised areas): £200–£400

Risks: loss of colour; sun-sensitivity; scarring

Length of stay in hospital: none

Anaesthetic: general or local

Other drugs: painkillers

Discomfort levels: high

Time before the signs of surgery disappear: three to six weeks

Length of time results last: semi-permanent.

LIGHT PEELING

Another less dramatic method is called light peeling, which is really a beauty treatment and involves using either a weak solution of TCA or one of the fruit acids – alpha hydroxy acids (AHAs). Fruit acids are commonly used in a very dilute form as exfoliants by the cosmetic industry.

Exfoliation loosens cells on the surface of skin so they slough off, revealing fresher smoother skin. It is said to increase the turnover of skin cells, plump up the epidermis, fade liver spots and increase production of collagen. However, to have any effect on the skin, there must be sufficient concentration of the acid but many creams and lotions contain only extremely dilute amounts.

Glycolic acid is a fruit acid derived from sugar cane and it is often used for light peeling, which consists of a course of four to six shallow peels carried out every week or fortnight.

The mild solution is applied and left on according to how long the person advising you considers is best – a few minutes to overnight. A light peel should not cause visible scabbing and scaling, just some stinging, flushing and dryness. It is then boosted by the use at home of creams containing glycolic acid.

A course of light peels is supposed to make skin softer, more supple and more youthful-looking and help diminish the appearance of fine wrinkles and brown marks on the face, hands, forearms and the upper chest. But light peeling is a commercial beauty treatment so results are far from dramatic.

There have also been reports of sensitivity to light peels, which can apparently cause red blotches and scabbing. This is unacceptable for a beauty treatment which may have little positive effect on the skin and is carried out without medical supervision.

Glycolic acid peels should not be undertaken during pregnancy, nor should they be used on hypersensitive skin or skin affected by eczema or psoriasis.

WRINKLE FILLERS

It's hard to love our wrinkles and the idea of being able to smooth out the lines on our faces by applying some sort of DIY filler from the outside is extremely appealing –

especially to those who are not yet ready to go all the way and have surgery.

Unfortunately, there is, as yet, no true biological wrinkle filler. But, for the short term, injections of collagen or other substances can satisfy many people's desires to erase their lines and wrinkles.

COLLAGEN

Injections of collagen can instantly reduce the appearance of nose-to-mouth grooves, frown furrows, acne pits and depressed scars and it can be used to enhance narrow lips (*see page 63*). A dilute form can also be used around the eyes.

Its effectiveness can be judged by the fact that it's one of the most popular cosmetic procedures, second only to lipo-suction in the US, where more than 2,000 faces are injected every week.

What is collagen? It's a protein that is the main constituent of skin, bones, muscles and ligaments. Fibres of collagen are interwoven throughout the dermis, acting as the skin's scaffolding. It weakens and disappears through-out a lifetime of smiles, frowns, smoking and exposure to sun, so tiny crevices appear in the dermis, causing the lines and wrinkles we see on the skin of our faces.

Cosmetic surgeons use a purified form of collagen retrieved from cowhide. It has been treated so that it is less likely to provoke an allergic reaction and it comes suspended in saline as a creamy white paste which can be easily injected into the crevice in the dermis.

As soon as it is injected, most of the saline is absorbed by the body leaving the collagen in place. Two to three outpatient treatments, two weeks apart, may be required to fill the crevice and smooth out the wrinkle.

Because collagen is a foreign protein, there is always the possibility of an allergic reaction. Around 3 per cent of people who have collagen injections will develop localised reactions – hard, red, itchy blotches which may take six months to disappear and may need treatment with steroids. So beware.

The surgeon should always ask if you have a history of allergy. People with rheumatoid arthritis should not have collagen injections.

A trial injection in the arm should be given as an allergy test a month ahead of treatment, although not everyone who is sensitive to collagen will react to the test. With any foreign protein injection there is a risk of anaphylactic shock – a potentially fatal allergic reaction affecting the whole body, including the heart and lungs. It is this risk that makes some doctors reluctant to use collagen. The cost of regaining a youthful appearance may be higher than you thought.

Treatment can be painful, especially when collagen is injected into the lip. An anaesthetic cream can be applied to the area prior to injections and a local anaesthetic – lignocaine – is mixed with the collagen.

There may be some swelling which can be flattened by rolling with a finger. Redness and bruising may last up to a couple of days. If the collagen has been injected too deeply, it will not show up. If too much collagen has been injected superficially, it can form a small ulcer, which may leave a mark. You may apply make-up after a couple of hours.

Collagen works very well in the short term for frown furrows at the top of the nose, for nose-to-mouth grooves and for the bracket marks caused by smiling. However, it's an expensive option in the long term, because it's absorbed into the body after three to six months, so you need to go back for top-ups, two or three times a year or more. Many men and women are happy to do just that, viewing the procedure as little different from having their hair coloured or their legs waxed.

'I started having collagen injections when I was 43,' says Diana Morgan, a solicitor who's now 47. 'I'd lost a bit of weight and my face had got thinner, so I decided to have collagen injections in the lines which run from my nose to mouth.

'It's not a pleasant procedure, it brings tears to my eyes. It leaves my skin a bit red and then I have to sort of roll it. But I look better instantly. The collagen's excellent at plumping out my face but it does wear down in three to four months – and that's the trouble.

'If I have it done three times a year, say, then I've had around a dozen sessions and the cost mounts up. As a result, I have had to shop around for it and some of the doctors I've tried have really made me look a mess.

'One doctor I saw before a holiday left me with great red marks from nose to mouth which took a week to fade. I do bruise easily, but how much depends entirely on the doctor's skill.

'I'm thinking of having a face-lift and my eyes done now. So you could say that all that collagen has been a complete waste of money. On the other hand, it has given me an extra few years before I go all the way with surgery.'

See page 88 for treatment details.

FAT

There is no evidence as yet that fat can be successfully harvested from one part of the body and injected somewhere else. It is reabsorbed by the body just as speedily as collagen, so it's not really any better, in that sense. Nevertheless, because it comes from your own body, there are no potential problems of a serious adverse reaction against it.

The fat is drawn out of the body (usually the abdomen) by liposuction (*see page 138*) and then injected into the wrinkles. This causes fat cells to break down into oil, which is then perceived by the body as foreign, and there is reaction around it, producing scarring. This is why it takes time to disappear.

SILICONE

Silicone, although foreign to the body, does not produce much reaction. However, it is often injected as a mixture with paraffin, which causes a reaction and therefore scarring. The scarring stops the silicone moving in the tissues.

In addition the body will attempt to reject the foreign substances and so silicone often ulcerates its way to the surface. To complicate matters further, the injected silicone puts pressure on the surrounding tissues so your own fat breaks down and gets absorbed, leaving even less padding than before.

All of these factors mean that injected silicone can become so hard and lumpy that it requires surgical removal – causing more scars. There also remains the unresolved question of its link with the development of autoimmune disease in women who have had silicone breast implants (*see page 109*), which many doctors dispute. This controversial issue led to its use as a wrinkle filler being banned in the US in 1992, although it is still available in Britain.

Silicone may work better as a solid facial implant. Prior to its ban in the US, surgeons had begun experimenting with the use of slivers of silicone inserted beneath the skin to smooth away laughter lines and nose-to-mouth grooves. The slivers are inserted through an incision inside the nose.

GORE-TEX

The main advantage to using Gore-Tex, which is used to make hiking gear weatherproof, is that it won't deteriorate over time, so results are permanent, unlike fat or collagen injections. Tiny strips of Gore-Tex are implanted beneath the epidermis in a process called threading. This can work well, because the strip gradually gets surrounded by scar tissue, plumping up skin by as much as 60 per cent to diminish fine lines.

Gore-Tex is non-allergenic, it doesn't cause autoimmune reactions and it can be shaped for the chin, cheeks or jaw line. It can also be used to enhance thin lips (*see page 63*), but has the same complications as silicone.

For instance, there have been reports of infection caused by the Gore-Tex, which can be difficult to treat and disfiguring, because the strips then have to be cut out of the skin. The Gore-Tex can also become displaced and the scarring round it can become so thick and fibrous that the skin feels extremely hard – which is a particular problem in lips.

Cost (collagen treatment): £110 for initial consultation and test and then £250 per ampoule

Risks: localised allergic reactions; lumpiness

Length of stay in hospital: none

Anaesthetic: none

Other drugs: none

Discomfort levels: low

Time before the signs of surgery disappear: no surgery, so no signs

Length of time results last: from a week to several months

CHAPTER SIX

More Ways of Dealing with the Skin

LASERS

The latest fix for problem skin is the use of lasers – high energy beams of intense light. Lasers have revolutionised the treatment of particular skin blemishes and they are now being used as tools to resurface the entire ageing face, replacing dermabrasion or peeling.

Lasers have been used in medicine since the 1960s and there seem to be no long-term dangers of their use. Some of the older types of laser could cause burns because it was hard to control their degree of penetration.

But today, in expert hands, they are extremely safe, they can produce good results and they create little or no scarring. So their cosmetic appeal is obvious. And they are now being tested for use on the neck area, on stretch marks and even as a method of hair removal.

The extent to which lasers penetrate the skin depends on the kind of laser used by the surgeon. There are several different types of laser producing beams of different colour and energy, which are selected according to the blemish being removed.

The colour of the beam depends on the chemical dye through which the particles of light pass and the wavelength of the light. The red, longer wavelengths penetrate the skin more deeply than the short violet ones.

The energy of the beam varies: continuous lasers are low energy and on all the time. Pulsed lasers are very high energy with intervals between pulses. A combination of selecting the right wavelength and pulse allows lasers to deliver energy faster than the surrounding tissues can conduct the heat, so they are not damaged. The Q-switched ruby laser, for instance, delivers light in nanoseconds (a nanosecond is a thousand millionth of a second), so that the melanin in liver spots is destroyed without any harm being done to the other layers of skin.

Ruby lasers are used to treat brown marks, such as liver spots, dark circles under the eyes and freckles, and also tattoos. The yellow-pulsed dye laser is used to treat red marks, such as port-wine stains, spider veins and also warts. The most versatile laser of all is the new carbon dioxide laser with a skin resurfacing attachment such as Ultrapulse or SilkTouch, which is used to treat fine lines and wrinkles.

How lasers work

The carbon dioxide laser vaporizes the treated surface before much heat can be conducted to the lower layer of skin. The surgeon uses a computer pattern generator scanner to map out squares of skin each of which are treated in a few microseconds. On deeper lines around the mouth, for instance, the laser will be passed four or five times along the shoulders of the wrinkle. Each pulse removes a very fine layer of epidermis, just a few cells thick. The heat that does reach underlying skin actually appears to shrink collagen (the skin's scaffolding) and promote the production of connective tissue, so skin becomes tighter and smoother. A recent study looked at 100 patients with different degrees of photo damage (the fine lines and wrinkles caused by exposure to the sun), who received treatment with the new carbon dioxide laser. They all showed some improvement as the skin regenerated, although this was not always obvious early on. But improvements continued up to 12 months later.

The risks

The carbon dioxide laser is extremely accurate to use. The surgeon can see very precisely how deep he or she is going and the risk of going too deep is small.

In general, the side effects of laser resurfacing are con-sidered to be less troublesome than from chemical peeling and dermabrasion. There is no charring or bleeding, just severe inflammation, like a bad case of sunburn. There is also no bleaching of the skin – if anything, skin becomes a little darker. However, like dermabrasion and peeling, a laser cannot erase deep furrows, although it can be targeted with great precision on deeper lines and wrinkles.

The major disadvantage of laser resurfacing is that the redness produced lasts for so long – a good three to four months. Laser treatment may also encourage a flare-up of the herpes virus, so a low dose of acyclovir should be started a day before treatment and continued for eight days after-wards if you have had this infection before.

Hospitalisation is not required for laser treatment and anaesthesia is not necessary for the ruby and yellow-pulsed lasers – except for children. Children having large coloured lesions, such as portwine stains, removed will be given a general anaesthetic as a day case. For some treatments, you will be given anaesthetic cream to rub in beforehand. Only local anaesthesia is needed for the carbon dioxide lasers unless the face is being completely resurfaced in which case you will be given a general anaesthetic as a day case.

Despite the advertising hype, the results of laser treatment cannot be guaranteed. The response of skin to a laser varies from person to person and not everyone is a good candidate for laser therapy. Not every clinic will have these lasers as they are extremely expensive.

TOTAL SKIN RESURFACING

You will be asked to arrive an hour ahead of your treatment in order to have anaesthetic cream applied to your face. You will be given a sedative and local anaesthetic will be injected into sensitive areas around the lips and eyelids. If you are very anxious a light general anaesthetic will be used. You (and the nursing and medical staff) will wear a special shield over your eyes.

Treatment of the whole face (right up to lips and eyelashes) takes around an hour and a half and is often done under general anaesthetic. Pain will take up to 24 hours to disappear but you will be able to go home 4 hours after treatment. But you will look dreadful – like a very severe sunburn victim, as your face will be swollen and your skin red. You will be given special cream to apply and antihistamine tablets to soothe any irritation, so you can sleep. What's more, you will look even worse for the next eight to nine days with red, raw, weeping, peeling skin and a swollen face.

Just over a week later you can apply some light

camouflage make-up. In the third week, you may look wonderful – because the residual swelling will make your new skin look as though it is completely wrinkle-free. In the fourth week, however, wrinkles will start to show up again.

However, over the next few months, your skin should continue to show improvements. You will be advised to use a sunscreen every day to protect your skin from further UV damage.

PORTWINE STAINS, BIRTHMARKS AND MOLES

These are areas of skin where there is extra pigment or enlarged blood vessels. Previous methods of treatment included surgery, freezing and radiotherapy, but now lasers are the treatment of choice – a ruby laser for dark birthmarks and a yellow-pulsed dye laser for red ones. Patients describe the sensation of the ruby laser as similar to the ping of having a rubber band snapped against skin. The yellow-pulsed dye laser has more of a dull thudding sensation. Patients often require more than one treatment – spaced by six weeks.

LIVER OR AGE SPOTS

These are round flat brown areas of skin which doctors call solar lentigos and we should call sun spots. They are caused by excess development of melanin (the pigment that darkens our skin to protect it from sunlight) on areas of the skin that are constantly exposed to the sun – the face and throat, the hands and the forearms. They can be frozen off with liquid nitrogen (cryosurgery), but it is difficult to be precise and overtreatment is common, resulting in white patches. Treatment with a ruby laser is the method of choice today – although if they are very superficial and light in colour, they can also be removed by a chemical peel or Retin A cream (*see page 96*). The skin must then be protected with a sunscreen.

'I grew up in the sun and I think that's why I developed some small liver spots on my cheek and forehead,' says Rosemary Sutcliffe, who's 49 and used to be a model. 'I was particularly bothered by one on my cheek which seemed to be getting larger and darker. So I asked my cosmetic surgeon to use the laser on them. I had to wear goggles, but I didn't need an anaesthetic. It didn't hurt – it's just like being smacked with an elastic band – and it only took five minutes.

'Afterwards the marks looked purplish and burned and an hour or so later, my face felt as though I'd been badly sunburned. I was given aloe vera gel to put on and after a few hours my skin stopped burning.

'A week later, the skin crusted over and flaked off where the laser had been. I was told I could wear cover-up make-up after ten days, but I wanted to leave it to heal, and the areas just faded to normal.'

TATTOO REMOVAL

How successfully a tattoo can be erased depends on when and how you had the tattoo done and on its colour. Younger tattoos tend to be removed more easily and quickly than much older ones. And removing amateur Indian ink tattoos may be less predictable due to the differing depths of pigment. Five to ten sessions of laser treatment are required to remove a tattoo using a Q-switched ruby laser.

'I was 15 when I had an eagle tattooed on my right forearm and a panther on my left,' says Eric Stewart, a journalist who's now 39. 'My older brother was having one done and I went along with him. My mother didn't know where we had gone and was outraged when we got home.

'I was so proud of my tattoos at school and usually wore my blazer with the sleeves rolled up to show them off. It wasn't until I was in my twenties that I realised quite how much of a social stigma tattoos were. From then on I never used to reveal my arms and used to wear long sleeves on the beach and at the tennis club.

'I've wanted to get rid of them for ten years now, but I didn't think anything could be done to get rid of them except skin grafting. But then I began to read about lasers. And eventually I went to see a surgeon.

'He told me that because my tattoos were mostly black they would be fairly easy to remove, though it would take several sessions. I've only had one so far. I had to wear special glasses for the treatment, which lasted about 40 minutes and was done under local anaesthetic. It still hurt – a bit like an elastic band being snapped against the skin – but nothing like the pain of having a tattoo.

'After the scab dropped off the skin was fine and the tattoos have faded by about 30 per cent. In three months' time I can go back for more laser treatment.'

Cost: around £150 for a laser test and then around £300 for each small area treated.

RETIN A CREAM

This is a cream containing a derivative of vitamin A, called tretinoin. Its rejuvenation effect was first noticed by people using it to treat acne, who found that as their spots disappeared so their fine lines and wrinkles became shallower.

Daily use of the cream over six to 12 months or more has been shown to modify the fine wrinkles, blotchiness and age spots, which are now thought to be caused largely by exposure to the sun (photo damage).

Retin A cream reverses the ageing effects of the sun by increasing cell turnover. New skin cells multiply in the base of the epidermis and force their way up to the surface, causing dead cells to be sloughed off more rapidly. Retin A cream also seems to encourage the production of collagen, so the dermis becomes more springy and the epidermis is thinner and smoother.

However, this miracle is not achieved without side effects. As old cells are shed, skin reddens, dries out and starts peeling, causing local irritation and sun sensitivity. A sunscreen must be used after Retin A treatment.

On stopping treatment, skin remains improved for one to two years, especially if a maintenance dose of cream is applied twice a week. Retin A has been used to treat acne for the past 25 years and there seem to be no long-term problems. However, it is not recommended for everyone – it can aggravate eczema and enlarge spider veins.

Some people who use Retin A do not notice any improvement. Surgeons and dermatologists suggest this is because they cannot remember how their faces looked to start with, which is why it is so important to take photographs before and after treatment.

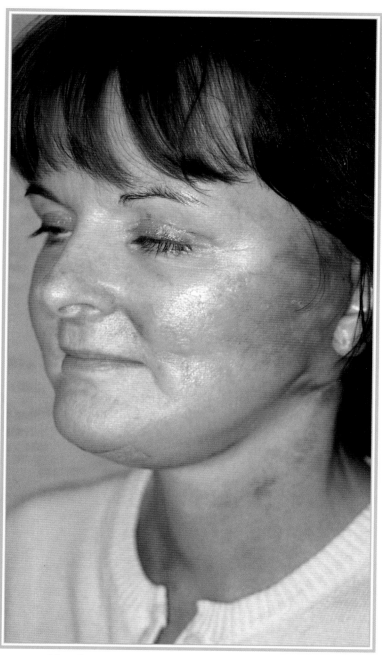

After face-lift and upper eyelid surgery, five days later

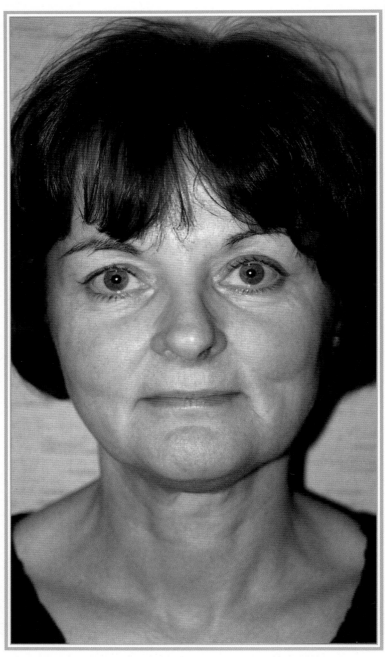

Before face-lift (extended SMAS) and upper eyelid surgery

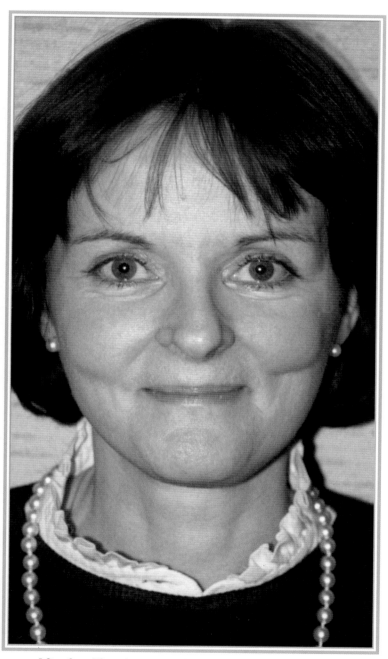

After face-lift and upper eyelid surgery, twelve weeks later

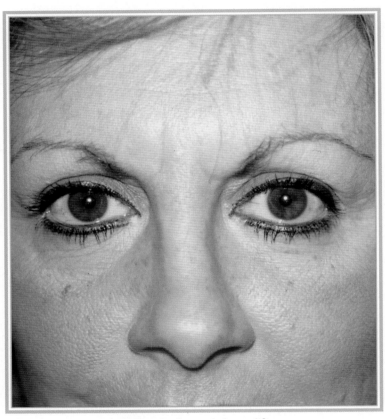

Before endoscopic brow-lift

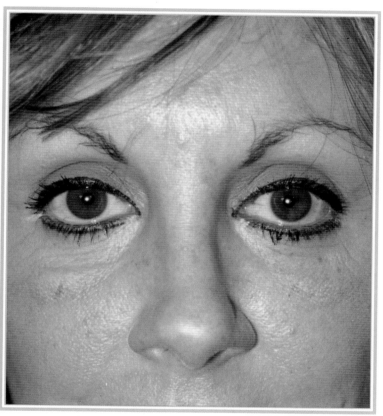

After endoscopic brow-lift, eleven weeks later

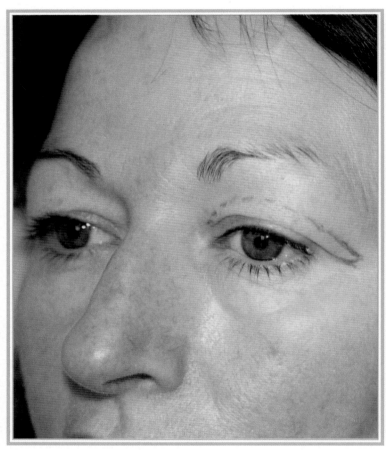

Before upper eyelid surgery

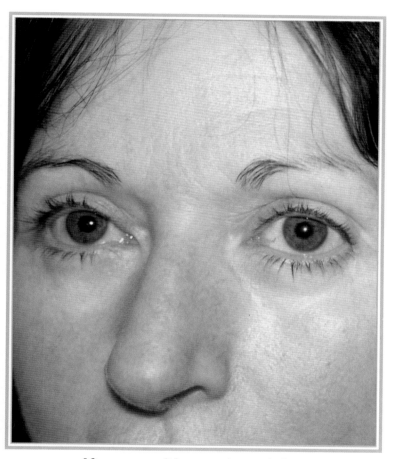

After upper eyelid surgery, ten weeks later

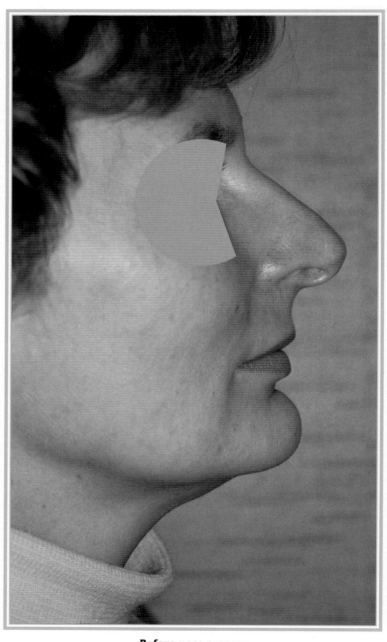

Before nose surgery

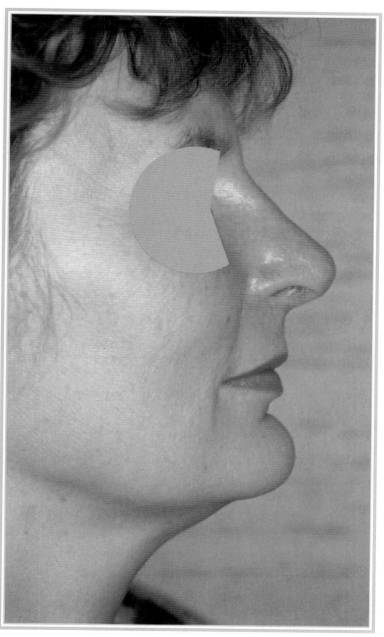

After nose surgery, twelve weeks later

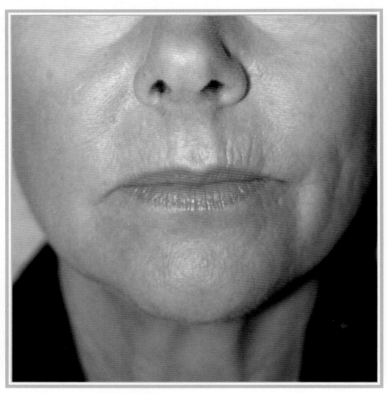

Before dermabrasion of the upper lip

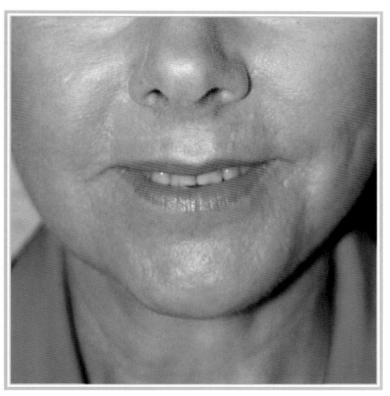

After dermabrasion of the upper lip, nine weeks later

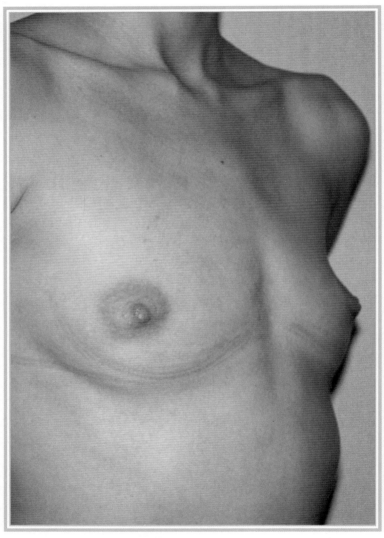

Before breast augmentation

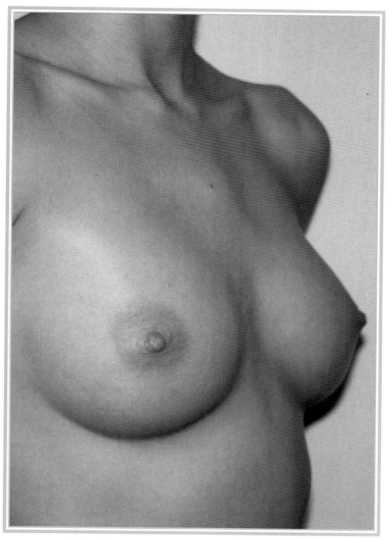

After breast augmentation, twelve weeks later

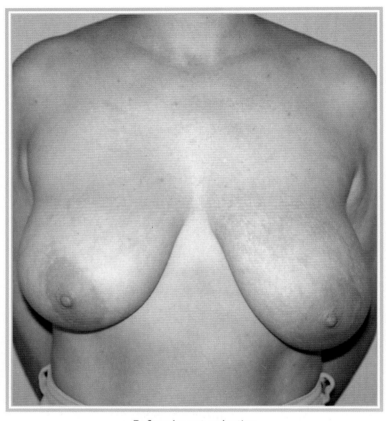

Before breast reduction

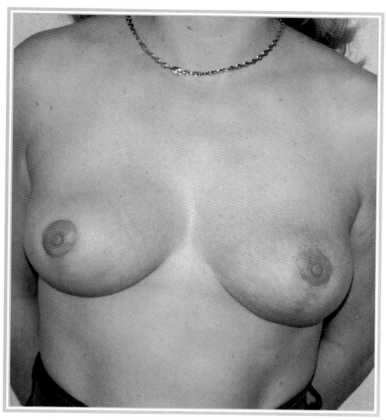

After breast reduction, twelve weeks later

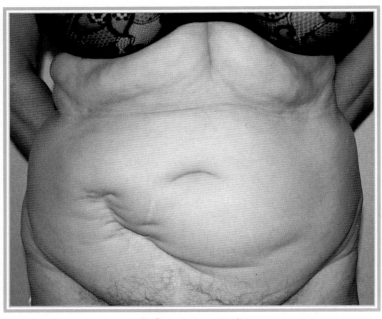

Before tummy tuck

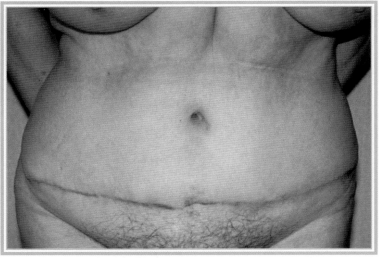

After tummy tuck, twenty weeks later

Retin A comes in three different strengths. The weakest is 0.025 per cent, the middle strength is 0.05 per cent and the strongest is 0.1 per cent. A recent study found that ageing skin responded just as well to the weakest strength cream.

Retinova is a new cream containing tretinoin, which has been fragranced and is greasier than Retin A in an effort to cut down its drying effects. It only comes in mid strength.

'I started using Retinova six months ago when I was coming up to my fortieth birthday,' says Nicola Jolly, a photographer.

'I could see wrinkles around my eyes, on my forehead and around my mouth and they bothered me. So I went to see a cosmetic surgeon, who said I didn't need surgery. My skin was just showing the beginning of sun damage, so he prescribed Retinova.

'After a week, my skin began to glow as though I'd been sitting in the sun. When I went out in the cold I could feel the wind and my face felt really tender. Then a couple of weeks later I started to peel on my forehead, at the corner of my lips and round my eyes, where I'd been putting the stuff. My skin looked and felt dry. I'd pile on the moisturiser in the morning and need more again by lunchtime. That lasted for about two weeks. But since then my skin has been fine.

'I noticed a difference around the lips in about a month. But I'm not sure if my eyes are better or not. Some days I think yes, some days no. On balance, I would say my skin has improved in look rather than actually getting rid of any lines. I'm on a maintenance dose now. Some nights I put it on, some nights I don't. I'm not really a very disciplined person. I did try putting it on the back of my hands and I thought they looked smoother, but I kept forgetting to do it.

'I've seen before and after photos which promise miraculous results with Retinova but that hasn't happened. On the other hand, those were all bad cases of wrinkles to start with and my face isn't that bad. I think that if I keep on with it, my skin will be better. It's going in the right direction. I want to do something, but nothing too dramatic – yet.'

Retinova is applied to clean skin once a day before going to bed. You may notice a feeling of warmth, some stinging and some skin flushing while applying it. You may use your own moisturisers and cosmetics in the morning and throughout the day – though you may find your skin more product-sensitive – and you are advised to use sunscreen as well.

After three months, improvements should start to show up. Once your skin is as good as it can be, you must continue applying the cream three times a week, otherwise the effects will wear off over time. The cream must not be used during pregnancy.

You can now obtain Retinova for sun-damaged skin on a private prescription from your GP or through a cosmetic surgeon or dermatologist.

'I've used Retinova on my face every night for around six months,' says Caroline Mansfield, who says she's over 60 and works as a picture-framer.

'I put it on all over after I've taken my make-up off (I never let water touch my face), and am careful to avoid going in close to the eyes. But I'm not totally impressed. It does work on the outer cheek areas, which don't look as cracked as they used to. But it doesn't work at all on the lipliner lines, in my opinion.

'I am always careful of going in the sun now I'm no

longer young. I cover up and wear lots of sunscreen because I know the sun is no good for my skin. I don't think I've suddenly become sun sensitive.

'I had incredibly high hopes of Retinova after reading about it, but it hasn't done much for me. People do tend to think that I'm in my early fifties, so maybe if I hadn't used it I'd look worse. But I really can't see much difference.'

Cost: Retinova, around £25 for a 20g tube, on private prescription, which lasts two to three months.

SPIDER VEINS

The medical term for red spider veins is telangiectasia. They are really tiny dilated capillaries. Their walls have lost their elasticity so they can no longer contract. They start showing up on cheeks, noses and legs as we get older – partly because the skin gets thinner with age.

Sun, wind, saunas, alcohol, smoking, sitting cross-legged and hormonal changes (particularly in pregnancy and taking HRT) all aggravate them, though the tendency to develop them is probably inherited. They may also develop on the site of an injury, such as a broken ankle or nose. There are several methods of treatment.

The first is called sclerotherapy, where an irritant solution is injected directly into the blood vessel so its walls stick together. The needle used is no wider than a human hair and after the injection gentle pressure is applied. The chemical spreads through the tiny network, which then shuts down and disappears altogether over the next few weeks.

Sclerotherapy must be carried out by a trained nurse or doctor. It's not advised if you're pregnant, diabetic or on steroids. An anaesthetic cream applied half an hour before treatment dulls the pricking sensation. Don't have it done just before an important event, because it leaves little bumps, although they soon disappear.

Spiders should fade after one treatment, but sclerotherapy is rarely completely effective. You'll be asked to return for reassessment and possible repeat treatment six weeks later.

'I had a small whorl of broken veins on my cheek, odd little veins where glasses used to press on my nose and right on the tip of my nose and two tiny red dots by my mouth, which I used to conceal with blobs of make-up,' says Jennifer Hutchins, who's a 35-year-old beauty therapist.

> 'A surgeon tried to get rid of them with sclerotherapy. The whorl is still there, but the veins on my nose are much less noticeable and the two red dots have vanished completely. I'd say it was 50 per cent successful.'

The second method is electrolysis. A current is passed through a needle applied to the skin over the vein so that it is sealed off. Good results are not guaranteed. Electrolysis, which is available from most beauticians, can leave tiny pitted scars and even provoke a new crop of thread veins.

The pulse-dye laser is now the best treatment for any red blotch or blood vessel in the skin including spider naevi and spider veins. It is less successful for small blue veins.

'I have very fair skin and I don't like wearing make-up,' says Debbie Harding, who's a health journalist aged 42.

'I've always tended to get ruddy cheeks, but what bothered me was the spider veins around the base of my nose – which may have occurred as a result of having had a nose job when I was younger.

'I spoke to a dermatologist who had started using a pulse laser and he booked me in. The treatment was over incredibly quickly. I just felt a few sharp pricks, I was given some aloe vera gel to put on and was told the area might feel sore. Well, it came up bruised and swollen and it felt numb for a few days. Ten days later it was fine. All the veins have gone – and I'd love to get more done – if I could afford it.'

Cost: sclerotherapy, £85–£300 per treatment; laser therapy, around £200 per treatment; electrolysis, from £15 per treatment

SCARRING

You may have the idea that a cosmetic surgeon can carry out an operation on you and there will be no scars left – almost as though he or she has done a bit of invisible mending. This is, of course, not true. Surgeons do their best to hide their incisions in folds of skin wherever possible so that the resulting scar is concealed and there will be no tension on the scar.

But if you have been left with a disfiguring scar on your face as a result of an accident then the surgeon can help you, although what he or she can do is limited. If there is tension on the scar so it is pulling on your eyelid, for instance, then the surgeon can carry out some eyelid surgery to reposition the eyelid into its usual position – which will, of course, cause fresh scars.

If the scar is raised or depressed, then the surgeon can improve its contour by cutting it out, levelling it and restitching it. Sometimes a surgeon may use dermabrasion or occasionally chemical peeling to flatten surrounding skin. Occasionally laser treatment can be used to lighten scars. And finally, you can always camouflage the scar with make-up.

All scars improve with time. Twelve weeks after an operation it is normal for them to be red, hard and to vary with the weather – making people feel very disappointed with the results of surgery. But over a period of time, depending on your age above all, scars will soften, flatten, lighten in colour, stop itching and generally look better. The time taken for scars to mature ranges from six months in an older person and one and a half years in a younger child.

Occasionally a scar will become very red, raised and itchy. This is called hypertrophic scarring. If the scar continues to itch and increase in size after a year, then it is called a keloid scar. Keloid scarring is relatively common in black and oriental people, less common in white people – except redheads. The danger areas for the formation of keloid scars are the front of the chest, the shoulders, the neck, the face and the earlobes (after ear-piercing).

Keloid scars cannot just be cut out, because they will recur. Something has to be done to stop the collagen forming in the wound. There are four methods of tackling collagen formation. The first is the application of pressure – you may be advised to wear a special compression garment, or helmet for the head.

The second is to splint the keloid scar with soft malleable

silastic. The third is to inject steroids into the scar. And the fourth is to cut out the keloid and apply a dose of superficial radiotherapy. This last method is often used on the face, where the benefits of getting rid of an ugly scar outweigh the risks of radiotherapy.

Nothing can be guaranteed when it comes to treating keloids and you must discuss with great care all the pros and cons of the different treatments with your surgeon. Nothing will erase a keloid completely but careful treatment can leave you with a much flattened, paler scar.

PERMANENT MAKE-UP

Up to now, tattooing has been the only way to make make-up last for ever. It's done a lot in Asia and the far East, where vegetable dyes are tattooed around the eyes, often without anaesthesia. Few of us are prepared to take such a drastic step. But if you are fed up with applying eye-liner every morning, yet can't bear to be seen without it, you might consider a new solution – make-up that stays on for around four years.

You can have your eyes defined in grey, brown or black (not blue), your brows intensified with the same colours, which is helpful for people who have overplucked their eyebrows, your lipline highlighted with a natural skin tone (not red) or you can have a perfect beauty spot created anywhere on your face.

The technique involves injecting pigment through a fine vibrating needle into the most superficial layers of the skin. A local anaesthetic cream numbs the area and anaesthetic eye drops are also used, if necessary.

As the colour only penetrates 0.2mm deep, it fades with time – unlike a tattoo, which is much deeper. A mix of iron and titanium oxide pigment is used, which has a low risk of allergy and will not run. Small dots of colour, rather than a solid line, are injected to create the most natural look for lips and eyes. The procedure takes approximately half an hour per lid and is done under a local anaesthetic.

There may be some swelling, bruising and tiny scabs a day or two afterwards. You should wait a few days before wearing contact lenses or applying eye make-up. A touch-up is required a fortnight later to perfect and strengthen the result. Once it's done, no one will ever know. They'll know only that your make-up always stays put – at the end of the day, in the pool, in bed and even when you're in tears.

'I wear eyeliner on my lower lid all the time, I can't bear to be seen without it,' says Nathalie Hawthorne, who's 28.

> 'I'm a fitness instructor and I have to look good. But when sweat gets into my eyes and makes them sting, I rub them and often rub the eyeliner off, and when I next catch sight of myself I've got a dirty streak down my face. So I decided to get my eyes made up permanently. I paid £900 and it should last for four to five years.
>
> 'I had local anaesthetic injected into my upper and lower eyelids and drops in the eye to stop me blinking. It took the surgeon an hour and a half to do and afterwards my eyes felt bruised and sore and my vision was fuzzy because of the drops.
>
> 'All that anyone can see is a dark brown line beneath my lower lashes, which looks entirely natural because it's not a hard line, but there's also dots of colour injected above the upper lashes. I have so much more confidence

about myself now, because I know I always look my best, even when I've been working out or been in the shower. It's perfect for my job.'

Cost: eyeliner, around £950; eyebrows, £750; lips, £650

CHAPTER SEVEN

Improving Breasts

Too big, too small, too droopy or one bigger than the other – many women are distressed by the shape of their breasts, either the way in which they originally grew or how they have changed with age and child bearing. Breast remodelling – mammoplasty – can reduce, augment, lift or reshape the breasts.

Breasts are made up of milk-producing glands surrounded by fibrous connective tissue and fat. Everyone has different amounts of fat and glandular tissue, which is why women's breasts are so varied.

Each gland consists of 15 to 25 sections, called lobules, separated by connective tissue and each supplied with a duct to the nipple, so there are 15 to 25 openings on both nipples. The ducts grow in from the nipple, dividing and subdividing like the branches of a tree and ending in tiny milk-producing areas called alveoli. It is the glandular part of the breast that responds to the hormonal cycle.

The gland is surrounded by fat, which is what makes the breast stick out, and the weight of it is supported by ligaments which run from the chest wall to the skin. The pinky-brown area surrounding the nipple is called the areola. It is dotted with tiny lumps, oil-producing glands which keep the areola lubricated.

Every month, breasts go through a series of changes. Once an egg has been released from an ovary, the supply of blood and lymph increases. The breasts retain this fluid and swell up, feeling fuller and heavier. If the egg isn't fertilised, hormone levels fall and breasts return to normal.

If the egg is fertilised and there is an increase in oestrogen, then the blood supply to the breasts increases by half as much again, the glandular tissue increases and the fat stores grow. By the time the baby is born, breasts are about twice as big as usual. After weaning, the glandular tissue shrinks and breasts return to their original size, although they may feel softer and slacker. Some women find that after breastfeeding their breasts are like empty sacks.

Different shapes and sizes

Breasts come in all shapes and sizes and one is usually slightly bigger than the other. We are none of us symmetrical. Shape and size is determined by genes, by hormonal stimulation during puberty and by build. Artificial hormones, such as the Pill and HRT, also affect their size and, because they're made up of so much fat, breasts get larger and smaller when weight is gained or lost.

Once a woman has had her family, breasts tend either to get bigger or smaller and they start to droop. This is because the supporting ligaments have failed to contract after being stretched in pregnancy and lactation and because skin has lost elasticity with age. After the menopause, the glandular tissue shrinks and the connective tissue slackens.

In general, cosmetic surgery should only be carried out at a young age (teenagers) if the problem is a marked difference in size between the breasts or if breasts are extremely large.

Any of these conditions can cause a young woman to hide herself away and avoid all social contact. In such circumstances, breast surgery might then be carried out on a teenager but only if her GP and parents were all involved.

MAKING BREASTS BIGGER

Breast augmentation is carried out on young women who remain virtually flat chested, on women whose breasts have shrunk after pregnancy and on women whose breasts have dropped with age – unless the nipple hangs below the crease underneath the breasts, in which case an uplift operation is best. Breast augmentation can have a huge psychological impact on women who feel inadequate in bed, on the beach and even in the shops – where it can be hard to find clothes which fit properly.

Confidence can be restored by the insertion of implants, which make the chest wall stick out so that the breast tissue then sticks out more. Implants do not, in general, interfere with breastfeeding.

Having breasts enlarged has become extremely fashionable during the last ten years or so, when many more women – including models and media stars, such as Pamela Anderson, Paula Yates and, of course, Dolly Parton, opted to increase their breast size.

There is also a large group of women who receive implants as part of reconstructive surgery following breast removal (mastectomy) due to cancer (*see page 131*). And there is a small number who receive implants because of two rare developmental disorders – the first is when one breast fails to grow (Poland's syndrome) and the second is when the breasts grow into long thin tubes with a large nipple pointing downwards (tubular breasts).

Around 5,000 women in Britain are believed to receive implants every year, 60 per cent for cosmetic reasons. Following the silicone scare, the number fell, and a few women even had their implants taken out, but the number is rising again.

Are my implants safe?

All implants consist of a silicone bag with a filling inside it. There are four types of filling: soft silicone gel, saline (salt water), soya bean oil and hydrogel (made of cellulose) – the injection of free, uncontained fat or silicone into the breasts should never be carried out.

Silicone implants were introduced into the United States in 1962. Silicone gel has the best texture for implants and, up until recently, was used the world over in preference to saline. The gel has the same consistency as body fat, so the implant is soft and pliable and may allow natural movement.

However, a few years ago, a group of US lawyers dealing with medical negligence claimed a link between silicone implants and the development of breast cancer and birth defects in babies born to mothers with implants.

More recently, the same lawyers claimed a link between silicone implants and the development of connective tissue disorders, ranging from ME (myalgic encephalomyelitis or chronic fatigue syndrome) to rheumatoid arthritis, with symptoms ranging from severe fatigue and lymph node swelling to memory abnormalities. These were reported to occur between one and ten years after breast surgery and were most common in women whose implants had ruptured.

The fear was that silicone leaking out from the implants – silicone bleed – and migrating round the body might be triggering an autoimmune response, which is when the body's defence system starts to attack itself.

These claims resulted in a US ban on silicone implants for cosmetic purposes in 1992, even though the lawyers are now agreed that silicone implants have nothing to do either with the development of birth defects or breast cancer. Indeed, the evidence shows that women who have implants actually have a lower rate of breast cancer. However, the lawyers have maintained that there might still be a link with connective tissue disorders, despite 18 reports (looking at more than a quarter of a million women) to the contrary.

The latest study from Harvard University looked at nearly 400,000 women and confirmed that the risk of developing a connective tissue disorder for women with implants was very small. Researchers from the Mayo Clinic in Minnesota found that only five out of 750 women with implants developed a connective tissue disorder over eight years, a rate no higher than that among a controlled group of 1,500 women without implants.

A study carried out in Scotland had a look at over 300 women who had had implants over the past ten years – 40 per cent for cosmetic reasons and 60 per cent following mastectomy. Women who had had their breasts enlarged were compared with healthy women who had not, and the women who had had implants following a mastectomy were compared with women with cancer who had not had reconstructive surgery. Not a single case of connective tissue disorder was found in either of the groups.

The UK Department of Health has given silicone implants a clean bill of health and doctors in Britain have largely concluded that they are safe.

The manufacturers have always maintained that silicone is safe, even though antibodies to silicone have been identified in the body. Silicone is used all the time for joint replacements. It's also used as lubrication for syringes, so that we're all exposed to it, and diabetics, for instance, have a very high level of exposure to it, yet no sign of illness.

Nevertheless, rather than risk the cost of defending themselves in court against any of the 2.2 million US women and claimants overseas who have had implants, the manufacturers created a trust fund worth over $4 billion to pay damages to the many thousands of women claiming ill effects from their implants. While there have been one or two spectacular awards, not a dollar has actually changed hands. The manufacturers have filed for protection against bankruptcy and are appealing. No one knows yet what will happen.

Meanwhile the evidence in favour of the safety of silicone gets stronger all the time. It may not be completely inert and it is certainly possible to be allergic to it but now that the walls of implants are so much thicker and stronger, they are less likely to rupture – although they might wear out after 30 to 40 years. In addition, if an implant does rupture, the scar tissue built up around it will localise the silicone gel and keep it in the right place.

Alternatives to silicone

As a result of the silicone ban, US surgeons have been forced to use saline implants for cosmetic operations. The real problem with these is that the silicone bag holding the saline solution has a tendency to wrinkle because it is not completely full. These wrinkles show up through the skin of thin women and they weaken the bag itself, which is then vulnerable to rupture.

One in ten saline implants rupture and when that happens the breast deflates rapidly and removal is necessary. Salt water, however, is obviously not harmful to the body and will simply be absorbed and excreted.

A new alternative to saline and silicone is soya bean oil. It is called the Trilucent implant, because it is radiotranslucent, which means that x-rays are able to penetrate through it so that an effective mammogram is possible. Silicone implants interfere with x-rays, so if you have them, you must tell the radiographer when you have your breasts screened so that the mammogram can be taken from a special angle.

It is also believed that soya bean oil can be metabolised safely by the body if an implant ruptures – although no one really knows for sure and Trilucent implants are not permitted in the United States. There are only a few reports in medical literature about these implants, which are on trial in Europe where each one has been fitted with a tiny numbered electronic chip so doctors can maintain a database on them.

The hydrogel implant is also being tried out on an experimental basis in Europe. Another substance, polyethylene glycol (PEG), which is used in eyedrops and moisturisers and is also radiotranslucent, is being investigated in the US. In the event of a leak, PEG is quickly and completely excreted by the body.

Hardening of implants

The implants are inserted through a small cut in the skin and a larger one inside the body, where the surgeon creates a pocket for it beneath breast tissue or beneath the muscles of the chest wall. These cuts heal by making a scar. The scar in the skin will be small, but the scar inside the body is much bigger, running right around the implant.

Everyone heals differently. Some people develop scar tissue that is thin and soft, while others develop scar tissue that is thick and hard. Thick scarring around the implant leads to the formation of a hard fibrous shell or capsule – capsulation – which contracts and squeezes the implant into a hard ball.

Mild hardening may not be a concern, but rock-hard implants cause pain and make the breast stick up. Until about six to seven years ago, around half of all women who had silicone implants developed this hardening, which spoilt the results of surgery and meant that some of them had to have their implants removed.

One particular type of silicone implant did not cause hardening, because it was coated with polyurethane foam. But polyurethane breaks down in the body into a chemical which may cause cancer in animals, and so these implants were withdrawn in 1990.

Surgeons now know that using silicone implants with a textured surface gives better results, because the rough surface interferes with scar formation. With this type of implant, just 7 per cent of women will get hardening of the breasts three years after having surgery. So hardening can still happen.

'I never had any breasts and was called Two Backs at school,' says Anne Fairbank, a solicitor who's 30.

> 'I would never take my top off in front of anyone, because I used to wear highly padded bras which came with nipples

that I'd buy – at a price – from the States. Naturally, I hated swimming because I had to take the bras off.

'The only time I was ever proud of my figure – I used to be a gymnast and am over 5ft 9in – was when I was breastfeeding my two children. But once I'd stopped I was simply left with two bits of flab. Then my husband ran off with a woman with enormous breasts, so I swore that as I had the money I would have implants.

'I had the operation last May for a special price of £1,900. But there was never any discussion of what the surgeon would do and no before and after pictures. I only saw him a few minutes before surgery, when he simply drew some lines on me and said to leave it to him. I wasn't given any post-operative instructions either.

'Well, I'm a 34B now, instead of a 34 nothing. And that's wonderful. But, while the right breast hangs properly, the left one is hard and painful and has been right from the start, waking me up at night.

'It bled a lot after the operation, which was carried out via the armpits so I've got red scars which are very noticeable when I lift my arms – I work out a lot and go rock climbing. I would have preferred the surgeon to have operated from beneath the breast but this was never discussed.

'I'm not sure what to do now. The pain has gone and the hardness has improved too. The breast was rock solid, but now I can move it around. Ideally, I would like to have the implant out and put back between the muscle fibres, which is what another doctor I consulted advised. I don't want to have it out altogether. I'm much too pleased with my improved figure and should have had implants years ago.'

What is involved

There are different ways of carrying out a breast implant operation. The incision may be made in either the armpit, around the areola, or beneath the breast. The advantage of cutting through the armpit is that the resulting scar is rarely seen. The disadvantages are that it can be difficult to stop any internal bleeding; if the implant has to be removed, the surgeon will cut beneath the breast making another scar; plus there is a risk of tightness across the armpit down to the elbow (a blood clot in a superficial vein) and damage to a nerve causing numbness in the inner arm. The advantage of cutting through the areola is that the scar heals well but it may be visible. The disadvantages are that it gives poor access to the muscle; it may interfere with

3 incisions for breast augmentation

1. Periareolar
2. Submammary
3. Axillary

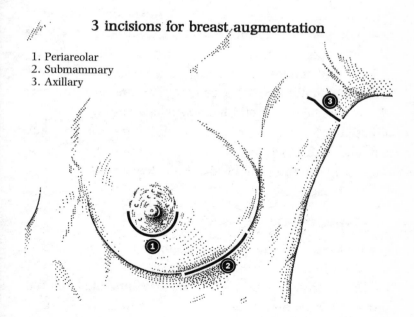

sensation in the nipple; and there's a limit to the size of the implant that can be inserted.

The advantage of cutting below the breast is that it gives good access; the disadvantage is that it can produce an obvious and ugly scar – however, some surgeons cut a little higher than the crease beneath the breast so that the scar does not show when you are lying on your back in a bikini.

The implant is placed either in front of the chest muscle or behind it. This has an impact on the subsequent shape of your breasts. Some surgeons prefer to place the implant in front of the muscle, which may work well to fill out a breast if it is an empty bag of skin.

If it is placed behind the muscle (against the ribs) then there will be more padding in front of the implant, so it is less likely to be felt.

The muscle forms a sleeve over it and the pressure against it may lessen the risk of encapsulation. The disadvantage is that when you flex your muscles the breast sometimes moves in a peculiar way.

Nowadays, endoscopic (keyhole) surgery may be used for breast augmentation, so the camera gives the surgeon direct vision. But he or she still has to make a cut big enough – about 5cm – to allow for insertion of the implant. By using saline implants, which are inserted empty and filled once they are in place, the cut need only be 2cm long.

Consulting a surgeon

If you decide to have a breast augmentation, the surgeon will want to find out a little about why you want it done. If you have only decided to do it because your husband has said he likes big breasts, it may be wrong to go ahead. If, on the other hand, you yourself feel lacking in femininity, then implants should restore your self-confidence.

The surgeon will take a full medical history, including any history of breast lumps or breast cancer, arthritis or neurological problems. If you do have arthritis, this doesn't mean that you can't have implants. The surgeon simply needs to know that the implants did not cause the arthritis.

Your breasts will then be examined and the position of each nipple will be checked. If they are too low then a straightforward augmentation is not the best solution. You'd be better off with a mastopexy (*see page 128*) as well.

The surgeon will look at your breasts carefully and measure them to check their symmetry – we're all asymmetrical, to a greater or lesser extent. But if your breasts are very unequal then it may be best to have different size implants to even them up. The surgeon will also feel for any lumps in the breast and armpits and check the skin tone and look for stretchmarks. Some people hope that breast surgery will remove the stretchmarks. It won't.

Bring along a bra that you would like to fill. It's no good saying you want to be a 36C or a 38B, because bra sizes are variable. Bring the bra and the surgeon will fit it with test implants for you to see.

There is a great variation in the price of implants. An average pair costs around £500, but you can pay up to £1,000. Implants range from 120ccs (small) to 450ccs (large). There are even larger ones available, as used by Dolly Parton.

Having the operation

When preparing for surgery, you should take no aspirin for two weeks and cut right down on smoking, stopping completely three days before the operation, to avoid any complications with the anaesthetic.

When you wake up from the operation, your new breasts will be taped in position with elastoplast. They will feel very sore, particularly if the implants were placed behind the chest muscle, which will be very bruised.

In general, it is best to stay in hospital for one night in case of pain. You will be discharged the following morning and you will be given painkillers (not aspirin) and anti-biotics, if necessary. A tube may be inserted to drain any fluid which might collect around the implant.

The pain will resolve in five to six days, and dressings and any stitches will be removed after ten days. You will also be asked to wear a Tubigrip around the chest or a special bra to hold the implants in the right place for a month after surgery. You should sleep on your back or side – not your front – for at least four weeks.

You can drive after ten days and three weeks after your operation you may resume gentle exercise. But violent movements and upward stretching of the arms is in-advisable for six weeks – so get someone else to wash your hair.

The risks

Complications of breast augmentation include infection, which is rare, and haematoma (accumulations of clotted blood) which need to be removed surgically. Much more common is a bad result, where implants are lopsided, with one breast higher than the other. The surgeon does the operation with you lying on your back but will often sit you up to try and ensure that your new breasts hang evenly.

Most women are completely comfortable with their new breasts and soon cease to be aware of the implants. However, everyone runs the risk of some loss of sensation in the nipples or elsewhere in the breasts. Some women actually notice increased sensation after implants. The bigger the implant, though, the more likely is the risk of nerve damage and loss of sensation.

The amount the breasts stick out afterwards – and the amount of cleavage – is impossible to predict. This is because the profile of your new breasts depends on how you scar around the implant – and everyone is different. It also takes time for scar tissue to develop – anything up to six months and more.

The textured silicone gel implants often feel quite hard at first and then soften up. There is no evidence that massaging the breasts stops the formation of the thick fibrous capsules. Some women are not unhappy with a degree of encapsulation, since it makes breasts stick out. But rock-hard breasts are painful.

It is not always obvious that an implant has ruptured. Any pain with a change of shape in an augmented breast should be investigated using ultrasound – the use of extremely high frequency sound waves to build a picture of what's going on inside the body – and mammography (x-rays).

Surgeons sometimes try to snap a capsule that has formed by squeezing the breast, hoping not to break the implant at the same time. This painful procedure is called a closed capsulotomy and should be rarely performed.

An operation to remove the old implant and the scar tissue around it is often necessary. Implant removal tends to leave a rather flattened breast, because the fat tends to waste away, so a replacement implant may be desired. Depending on the thickness of the capsule, the surgeon may recommend its removal at the time of replacing the implant. This is a bigger operation because there is the possibility of bleeding from the raw surface. In addition, if you want implants removed because you are worried about the dangers of silicone, there is no guarantee that it will reduce your risk of developing a connective tissue disorder.

Breasts should continue to be examined regularly for lumps and you must inform the radiographer that you've got implants before having a mammogram. Women on HRT should also be checked regularly using ultrasound and mammography.

A late complication of breast augmentation is when the breast continues to droop and the implant is left high up – so the nipple is below it. This must either be accepted, or the implant must be removed and repositioned, or you can have an uplift operation (*see page 128*).

'I was 41 when I decided to have my breasts enlarged. I'd started to get much bigger around the hips and my small breasts made me look unbalanced,' says Harriet Black, an administrator who's now 49.

'So I had the op after lengthy discussions with my surgeon. I had a face-lift at the same time, so I felt pretty dreadful after surgery. But I never felt any pain in my breasts. There was a little wound in my armpit and my breasts were taped down.

'When I finally saw them for the first time, I was thrilled. They'd gone from a 34B to a 36C and they were lovely and firm. Of course, being implants, they don't lie down flat the way natural breasts do, but I like that. And

I'd thoroughly recommend the op to anyone who's unhappy about having small breasts.

'I'm slightly concerned now that I'm coming up to the time for having mammograms, but I'm not bothered enough to change the silicone for the ones which are OK with x-rays. Why disturb something that's absolutely fine?'

Cost: around £3,000 to £3,500

Risks: capsule formation; asymmetry; loss of sensation in the nipples

Ideal age: late teens to late forties

Length of stay in hospital: one night

Anaesthetic: general

Other drugs: painkillers and antibiotics

Discomfort levels: high

Time before the signs of surgery disappear: four weeks

Length of time results last: permanent

MAKING BREASTS SMALLER

The aim of a breast-reducing operation is to create a natural shape and to retain function and sensation in the nipples as much as possible.

Large breasts attract a lot of unwanted attention and can be difficult to disguise. Women with large breasts are relentlessly singled out by men who view their breasts as exclusively sexual objects, which causes extreme self-consciousness and distress. Surgery not only can bring enormous psychological relief, but it relieves the physical distress of large breasts, too.

There may be pain in the breasts as well as other physical problems – they interfere with sport and exercise, they cause backache, skin problems can develop beneath them, weals can develop across the shoulders where bra straps cut in and their sheer weight means that they will hang lower and lower, causing skin to stretch and lose its elasticity.

Large breasts can develop in youth. This condition, called virginal hypertrophy, occurs when breasts are so sensitive to the hormone oestrogen that they simply balloon in size and can end up weighing as much as 4–5kg each.

Extremely large breasts can also just keep on growing so that they are oversized by the time a girl is in her late teens or early twenties. They can get bigger after pregnancy and they can continue to enlarge after the age of 45. Another reason for surgery is when there is a great difference in size or shape between the two breasts.

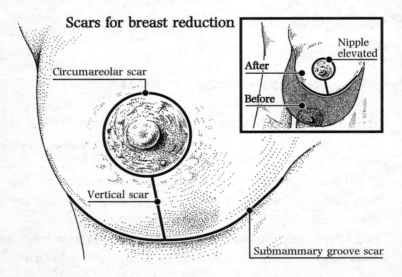

Scars for breast reduction

Circumareolar scar

Nipple elevated

After

Before

Vertical scar

Submammary groove scar

Having your breasts reduced is a major operation, but it causes surprisingly little pain and only requires one night in hospital. It can, however, cause bad scarring, depending on the individual and if stitching is poor.

Most scars will fade with time – and these scars are usually hidden. A few younger women do develop red unsightly (keloid) scars, but this is unusual and can often be helped.

What is involved

The surgeon will carefully measure and mark out the breasts with a marker pen, according to the size you want, which you will have discussed before.

Once you are asleep, the nipple – on a bed of tissue and still attached to its blood supply – is moved to its new, higher position, usually at the level of the crease underneath the breast. Then the lower part of the breast is removed to make it smaller. (Modern techniques mean that a blood transfusion is rarely required.)

Cutting through the dense tissue of young breasts is a little like cutting a pear, but in the older patient, when there is much more fat in the breast, this fat may be removed with liposuction (*see page 138*). The fold of fat in the armpit – which may be a supernumerary breast – is also sucked out.

The skin is then tailored, cut back over the new breast and stitched, leaving three scars: one around the nipple, one running from the nipple to the crease below the breast and one long one from the breastbone to the armpit along the crease below the breast. These scars should not be visible outside a bra or bikini top.

When the nipple is repositioned, it should still function and have normal sensation. However, some feeling may be lost to start with, but it should come back after three months. In very large-breasted women, where moving the nipple is more diff-icult, it is completely cut away and repositioned as a skin graft.

Breastfeeding may be possible after breast reduction, although it is better to postpone the operation, if possible, until after you have had your family, as pregnancy and breast-feeding will enlarge your breasts and cause them to lose their new shape. If you have had your nipples cut away and grafted into their new positions, you won't be able to breastfeed.

A common surgical error is to reposition the nipple too high, so that when the breast slips down with gravity, the nipple is left stranded.

Worse still, the nipple does not always survive the surgery and will partially or completely die. There is an increased risk of this if you are a smoker, are overweight, have poor circulation or breathing difficulties.

'I was 58 when I had my operation,' says Sarah Partridge, who's a librarian, 'and extremely large. I'd got bigger and had gone up from a 38D to a 38G and I'm only 5ft 2in. My bra straps were cutting right into my shoulders, which were beginning to bleed.

'I went into hospital at midday on the Monday, had the operation at 2pm and was out on the Wednesday. There was no pain or bruising at all. The only thing was that I was allergic to elastoplast so that was painful.

'I have scars underneath both breasts and around the nipples, but over the months they have faded. Now I'm a 38C/D and it makes such a difference. My shoulders are better and I'm delighted with my figure. It's the best thing I've ever had done.

'I always spent a lot on clothes to disguise how big I was, but now I can wear different clothes and I'm much more confident. My husband is pleased, it was his Christmas present to me. But he loved me as I was. I really had it done for myself. I only wish I'd done it earlier.'

Consulting a surgeon

If you seek a reduction, the surgeon will take a full medical history, including any family history of breast cancer. Your breasts will be examined carefully for any abnormalities, such as cysts or, in the older woman, cancer.

During the consultation, there should be a full discussion of scarring and how impossible it is to predict how good or bad your scars will be. You must also discuss together the size of breasts you eventually want to have.

'I was 24 when I had it done, in time for my wedding,' says Jane Ashby, who had a single breast reduced because it was larger than the other – a surprisingly common problem.

'I'd been squashing that one breast into a bra cup 38C/D, which was far too small, and wearing round necks and polo necks to cover myself up. I had found it hard at school and always hated swimming – I would never dream of going topless. I had never been a believer in cosmetic surgery, but when I spoke to someone with the same problem who'd noticed the difference get worse when she was pregnant, I decided to get my breast reduced. Of course, I could have decided to have the other one enlarged, but I didn't want big breasts.

'Now I have a scar from the nipple to the underside that still shows, but the scar around the nipple has virtually disappeared. I'm a balanced 38B and the difference to my life is really amazing. For the first time I'm wearing feminine clothes and my whole posture has changed.

'I never even realised before that I was slouching, but people at work actually asked if I'd had my shoulder fixed. I haven't lost any sensation in my nipple. And my fiancé's delighted. He wasn't bothered before, but he's just pleased because I feel so much better about myself.'

Having the operation

Before surgery, you should take no aspirin for two weeks and cut down smoking, stopping completely three days before surgery. The operation itself lasts two to three hours and you will wake up with drains from the breasts which will be removed the following day, when you should be able to leave hospital.

You need to bring a bra with you to support your new breasts. To make sure you're left with only the finest possible scars, you will be shown how to dress your cuts, once they are healed, with micropore tape for the first six weeks.

You must avoid stretching the scars and so all unnecessary activity of the shoulders and arms should be avoided. You will probably need two to three weeks' convalescence before returning to work.

The risks

Complications which may arise after the operation include the development of collections of clotted blood (haematoma), which may have to be surgically removed. These clots may resolve on their own about two weeks later, when a brown fluid is discharged from the wound, often when you're having a bath

At the point where the vertical scar joins the horizontal one, it is common to get some skin dying off. There is no specific treatment for this and it usually heals by itself in two to three weeks.

Very occasionally, there may be partial or complete loss of the nipple. It may go pale in which case its colour can be touched up later by tattooing. A major but rare complication is if it dies off completely. If this happens it is possible to make a new one later (*see page 136*).

In around three out of 100 cases, some of the fat inside the breast dies off in reaction to the surgery. This causes the breast to become red and hot. Eventually, there may be a discharge of brown fluid from a scarline and there may be lumps afterwards, which can be removed at a later date if they are a worry.

Most common of all is bad scarring and lopsided breasts. The vertical scar is the one which causes most problems because it takes most of the tension of the operation. But time, rather than treatment, is what is required for healing.

Every woman's breasts droop with age and, eventually, they will start to droop after surgery – even though they may start off plump and firm. They may also get a little smaller as the fat shrinks.

The latest surgical improvement aims to reduce the scarring caused by this operation by leaving out the horizontal cut. The stitches are placed under the skin on the gland tissue to shape it after reduction. The skin is then draped over the reduced breast in the hope that it will contract naturally.

This should work for younger women with good skin tone whose breasts were originally not too large. It takes time for skin to contract and you will be advised to wear a bra day and night for three months. If the skin does not contract, you can have it reduced later in a minor tailoring operation, done under local anaesthetic.

Cost: around £3,500

Risks: loss of sensation in the nipple; nipple loss; inability to breastfeed; fat loss; blood clots

Ideal age: late teens to old age

Length of stay in hospital: one to two nights

Anaesthetic: general

Other drugs: mild painkillers

Discomfort levels: mild to medium

Time before the signs of surgery disappear: 12 weeks

Length of time results last: permanent

PERKING UP BREASTS

After pregnancy or weight reduction, the breasts often change. In some women they go back to how they were before, in others, the glands shrink but not the skin, which causes sagging. If a woman desires uplift, with no increase in size, then this operation – called a mastopexy – is the one she wants. It is usually done as a day case under general anaesthesia.

The aim of surgery is to reposition the nipple, pull up the breast tissue and reduce the amount of skin. The design of the operation is based on a breast reduction, with similar scars – although often without the long scar in the crease below the breast. The complications are the same as for a breast reduction, but because less has been done, all the risks are much lower. It is very rare to have any problems with nipple survival and unusual to have any fat dying off.

As the operation aims to lift up the glandular tissue, you may be left with a tight vertical scar which, at first, may make the breast look very square and flat below the nipple. This takes time to settle and you will be advised to wear a particularly supportive bra.

When you first consult the surgeon, your breasts will be examined and the position of your nipples will be checked. If they lie below the crease beneath your breasts and you feel your breasts are too small, you will be advised to have a mastopexy with implants as well. Nowadays, these are increasingly being inserted during the mastopexy, but they can still be added at a later date. Doing everything at once can be a difficult operation because of the combined risks of breast augmentation and breast reduction.

A mastopexy should not be done if you are likely to have more children.

'I've had three children with the last pregnancy complicated by high blood pressure and putting on a vast amount of weight,' says Jean Symmons a busy mother aged 36.

> 'When I finished breastfeeding, I was left with breasts like empty sacks with my nipples almost down to my tummy button. They were like spaniel's ears and I felt really self-conscious. So I decided to go for surgery.
>
> 'I was amazed when the surgeon told me I needed

implants and that the nipple would have to be lifted up. I'd imagined he could just have hitched the whole lot up with a tuck in the armpit.

'I went into hospital on the morning of my operation and the surgeon drew lines all over me. When I woke up, I had a lot of pain in my chest and tubes coming out from my armpits, but I could see that my breasts were back where they had been 20 years ago.

'I returned two weeks later and my dressings were removed to reveal my battered breasts. I was astonished at the extent of the bruising but I looked like a teenager again. Over the next few weeks the bruising disappeared and my breasts became softer.

'One year later, I feel so much more self-confident, particularly when I go to the gym. My nipples are in a slightly different position and one of them does not have particularly good sensation but this is a small price to pay for feeling so much better about myself.'

Cost: around £3,500

Risks: same as for breast reduction but all are less likely to occur

Ideal age: 40-plus, after children

Length of stay in hospital: none to one night

Anaesthetic: general anaesthetic day case

Other drugs: painkillers and antibiotics

Discomfort levels: low to medium

Time before the signs of surgery disappear: 12 weeks

Length of time results last: breasts will continue to droop with age

RECONSTRUCTION AFTER A MASTECTOMY

There has been a big change in the way breast cancer is treated and fewer women today have to suffer the mutilation of a complete mastectomy (removal of the breast). Standard treatment can consist of a lumpectomy (removal of the lump and, usually, lymph nodes in the armpit) followed by radiotherapy and/or chemotherapy.

Virtually anyone who has lost all or part of a breast due to surgery for cancer can have breast reconstruction on the NHS and, increasingly, it is being done at the same time as the removal.

What matters most for a woman at the time of a mastectomy is whether or not she will survive the cancer. So she may not seek reconstruction until later, when she has survived her cancer and becomes more aware of her body image and of the effect of her appearance on her partner.

A breast reconstruction can help a woman feel whole and well after her battle with a life-threatening disease. But services are patchy and not all women are offered reconstruction. However, many don't mind wearing an external prosthesis (dummy breast).

'My self-image was never very good,' says Cathy Brewer, who's 49 and a systems analyst. 'So at first I was determined not to have a mastectomy. But I had two days to decide what the surgeon should do and, as I talked to my husband and read around the subject, I realised that if I had a lumpectomy I would worry about the cancer coming back. I really didn't want radiotherapy.

'So I opted for a mastectomy and reconstruction. They removed the breast and 11 lymph nodes and inserted a

silicone-covered bag of saline with a valve in the side of
the breast. Over the next few weeks, I had three
pumping-up sessions so it grew bigger and stood straight
out. Then they drained it a little to give it some natural
droop and removed the valve.

'But it still looks like the breast of a 20 year old, so
they've offered me surgery on the other side to get a
better match. I now have a great cleavage and some
sensation still at the top of the breast. It's not a sexual
response and it feels different from the other one, but it's
part of me. The scar is very small and I don't have a
nipple, so I feel self-conscious when I go swimming. But
I'm thinking of having one constructed.'

What is involved

A breast may be reconstructed in a number of different
ways, depending on the type of mastectomy, breast size,
position of the nipple and whether or not a woman has had
radiotherapy, which affects the way skin heals.

If a woman has healthy chest muscle and good quality
skin then it may be easy for the surgeon simply to insert an
implant via the mastectomy scar into a pocket created
under the chest muscle. The implant is the same sort as
those used for breast augmentation and, in the US, surgeons
are permitted to use silicone implants for this operation. It is
sometimes possible to improve the look of a poor mastectomy scar at the same time.

If there is not enough skin to stretch over an implant, but
the skin left is of good quality, a surgeon may insert a
temporary tissue expander – an empty bag, which is filled
with saline and topped up with injections over the course of

12 weeks or so, until the skin has stretched enough (as it does during pregnancy) to accommodate an implant. This is finally inserted, under general anaesthesia as a day case, when the tissue expander is removed. If the breast on the other side is very large, it may be necessary to reduce it down to the size of the reconstructed breast.

If the patient has had radiotherapy, it will not be possible to stretch the skin so an implant with new skin will have to be introduced. Patients have the choice of having tissue transferred from the back or from the abdomen.

In the first method, called latissimus dorsi, a flap of skin and muscle from below the shoulder blade on the back is turned round and tunnelled through beneath the skin to emerge from under the armpit. It is then used to cover an implant.

The operation takes several hours, recovery several weeks and a scar is left on the back. The disadvantage of it is that the reconstructed breast is usually too firm and not droopy enough to match the other breast, so an uplift operation may be required on that one as well.

The most superior method of treatment is to create bulk for the breast from the woman's own fatty tissue, by taking skin, fat and muscle from the abdomen. This is a complex operation called TRAM (transverse rectus abdominus myocutaneous) flap.

The surgeon takes a large almond-shaped swathe of flesh from the belly and either removes it completely, rejoining it by microsurgery to arteries and veins in the armpit, or pivots it round and tunnels the whole lot up under the skin of the abdomen to bring it out on the chest wall, without severing the muscle that supplies the block of tissue with blood.

The fat transfer to the new breast allows for a truly

natural consistency and droopiness – which means that balancing surgery on the opposite breast is less likely to be necessary. But a TRAM flap is a major operation that takes around four hours to do and requires a long recovery time.

The risks

The pitfalls of breast reconstruction are asymmetry – in size, shape and position; failure of the skin flaps (which fail in up to one in ten patients); and weakness of the abdominal wall in the TRAM flap procedure. TRAM is not a true tummy tuck operation. Even though the surgeon will strengthen the tummy wall with plastic mesh, one in four women who have this operation will end up with a weakness in their abdomen. They may even develop a hernia – a painful condition where the gut bulges out through the muscle wall.

It takes a long time to recover from a TRAM flap reconstruction. But it is an alternative to implants, especially if a woman has had extensive radiotherapy, because it means that irradiated skin can be replaced.

Nipple reconstruction (*see page 136*) is usually done a few months later.

Cost: around £4,500 to £5,000

Risks: asymmetry; skin flap failure; weakness of abdominal wall

Ideal age: any age

Length of stay in hospital: a simple implant can be done as a day case; five days in hospital may be necessary for a major flap reconstruction

Anaesthetic: general

Other drugs: painkillers and antibiotics

Discomfort levels: high

Time before the signs of surgery disappear: they remain

Length of time results last: permanent

INVERTED NIPPLES

Some women have nipples that point permanently inwards, a condition called inverted nipples. Some women have nipples that point inwards from time to time – retracted nipples. Both these conditions are usually caused by a short milk duct pulling the outside of the nipple in.

There is a device called a Nipplette, available from any high-street chemist, which may help with retracted nipples but not inverted ones. When you place the Nipplette on the breast, it stretches the duct by suction. However, it usually has little more than a temporary effect and can cause ulceration on the nipple. So some women seek a permanent solution.

Surgery for inverted nipples must not be done until a woman has had her family since it prevents breastfeeding. The surgeon will always check first for a history or any signs of breast cancer, since inverted nipples are occasionally a symptom of cancer.

The operation is done under local anaesthesia and is mostly very successful. The surgeon cuts into the nipple and divides the ducts, inserting a stitch like a purse string around the base of the nipple so they don't rejoin. This does not usually interfere with sensation, but the condition can sometimes recur.

Cost: £250

Risks: recurrence; breast feeding impossible

Ideal age: any age but after having children

Length of stay in hospital: none

Anaesthetic: local

Other drugs: none

Discomfort levels: low

Time before the signs of surgery disappear: three weeks

Length of time results last: permanent

CREATING A NIPPLE

For many women who have had a breast reconstructed, the surgery is not complete until they have a nipple made. It is usually done six months after the breast operation, allowing time for the breast to drop down into position. During this period, a stick-on artificial nipple may be worn.

There are two ways of constructing a nipple. One is to shave off half of the nipple on the other breast and graft it on to the new one – easily done under local anaesthetic. This is a straightforward technique called nipple sharing and the shaved nipple heals in a week. The areola is tattooed on around the new nipple three months later.

Some women either have small nipples to start with, so there is not enough to share, or they don't want the other breast interfered with. In these cases, a nipple is created by cutting a T-shape into the skin of the new breast and creating a mound. Then the surgeon cuts a circle around the base of the mound and grafts on to it a piece of dark skin taken from the top of the thigh. This can be done under local anaesthesia or as a day case under general anaesthesia.

'I had a nipple constructed from a circle of skin taken from the top of the back of my thigh, just where a swimsuit would end,' says Gillian Bennett, a fashion buyer aged 43, who had a breast reconstructed after a mastectomy two years ago.

'The way the surgeon cut and folded this piece of skin on the reconstructed breast and created the actual nipple was so clever.

'But it's bigger than the other one and lighter in colour – too pink. Also, the scar around it where he stitched it on still shows, making a red outline of this pink funny-looking nipple. But he has offered to tattoo it a darker colour, which I think should do the trick.

'I know I'll never look natural again – I had to have the other breast lifted to match the reconstructed one, so that one's scarred too, although those scars healed really quickly. I don't walk around naked anymore but I look OK, especially in a bra.'

CHAPTER EIGHT

Body Contouring/Fat Removal

Wafer-thin models are the beauties of our age. But the drive to match up to such unrealistic slimness has created a generation of women who feel they are too fat and who try – and usually fail – to control their eating patterns. A healthy body is neither too fat nor too thin but somewhere in between. Body shape is largely inherited and can't really be changed. We may be long and thin, plump and round, muscular or a bit of a mixture.

Women need some fat for fertility. When a girl starts her periods and is ovulating, she will have laid down at least 17 per cent of her body weight as fat. The ideal body composition for women is around 22 per cent fat, with an acceptable range of 18 to 25.

Women store fat mostly on hips and thighs in a pear shape. Men have less fat which tends to be stored around and above the waist in an apple shape. For men, the ideal body composition is around 15 per cent fat with an acceptable range of 11 to 18.

Excess fat stored around the middle of the body is a risk factor for heart disease. And because we tend to lose weight from the head downwards, women can find it particularly hard to shift fat from their hips and thighs. Men can find it hard to lose weight from the waist.

When a woman's production of oestrogen falls in the run-up to the menopause, she starts to store fat in the male pattern around and above the waist. This is partly why a woman's shape changes with age.

In general, as we grow older, we all lay down more fat in our trunks, particularly inside the body, around organs but we lose fat from our extremities – such as our hands and forearms. There are also racial differences in fat accumulation: black people, for example, store much more fat in the buttocks.

Scientists used to believe that we were born with the same number of fat cells. These were either full or empty according to how many calories we took in and how much energy we used up. It's now believed that we start off with an individually programmed number of fat cells. If we take in more calories than we use up, then we fill the cells and they will enlarge. If we continue to take in more energy than we use up then we may be able to make more fat cells – but this only occurs when an individual is seriously obese, that is, more than double ideal body weight.

No one knows for certain whether fat cells disappear when we lose weight or whether they remain empty, waiting to fill up again. But the only sure way of getting rid of them permanently is by liposuction.

SUCKING OUT THE FAT

Liposuction is not a method of losing weight and is no substitute for diet and exercise. It is a means of removing stubborn deposits of fat which can't be shifted by diet and exercise, such as saddlebag thighs and love handles.

Liposuction – sometimes called suction lipectomy – is the

removal of fat by suction. It is the most common operation carried out in the United States, more common even than hernia repairs, and 300,000 liposuctions were carried out in the US in 1995.

The technique was popularised by a French gynaecologist who had the bright idea of using the cannulas (tubes) used to scrape out the womb to suck out body fat instead. He tried sucking out some fat from the knees of a well-known ballerina in 1921 but, tragically, she ended up having to have a leg amputated!

Today, liposuction is most successful when used on young, healthy women. But it may be used satisfactorily on middle-aged women who are within a stone of their ideal body weight and who have good skin tone. Skin should be elastic enough to contract after the fat has been removed.

Although the best results are obtained with the elastic skin of younger women, teenagers are likely to be disappointed because their expectations may be very high. Liposuction will not turn anyone into Kate Moss. It will not turn thick legs into thin ones and it should not be used to treat obesity.

Neither is it a good idea to use liposuction on adolescents because young women's weight often takes several years to settle down. If a woman has liposuction and then gains weight, she may well develop a lumpy shape because new fat cells may grow unevenly.

However, liposuction can be extremely successful at dealing with diet-resistant areas of fat – such as saddlebag thighs and love handles.

'I had my thighs done two years ago,' says Mary Anderson, who's 34 and a farmer.

'I was a little overweight, it's fair to say, but my huge fat

thighs were like those of a 20st woman. I have a thin face
and know how to dress to bring out my best points. I could
wear a size 14 around the waist. I simply never wore jeans
or trousers, never wore skirts above the knee and never
went swimming or riding. And I wanted to do all of those
things – particularly the sport, because I wanted to lose
weight.

'I'd always dreamed of having liposuction. When I
finally went to see the surgeon I think he saw my top half
and didn't really believe I needed it. I remember him
asking me why I wanted it but when he saw my legs, I
noticed the look of surprise cross his face. Then he said
something about possibly needing to have two goes.

'I woke up from the anaesthetic simply glad to be alive
and then felt rather sick. But there was no pain. My legs
were bandaged from knees to bum and there was a thick
nylon corset over that right up over my tummy. I felt fine
so I left hospital and went to stay with a friend who's a
nurse.

'After five or six days I was so hot in the bandages that I
cut them off. My legs were black and blue but they were
definitely slimmer. I could see tiny cuts by the knee and in
the front and back of the thigh. I put the corset back on
and wore it for a month or so, only taking it off for an
hour to wash and dry it quickly.

'I'm still a bit overweight and flabby. But I feel a
thousand times better about myself. I've stopped smoking. I swim every day, go to step and aerobics classes
three times a week and I've even bought myself a trouser
suit, which people say I look really good in – though of
course they never knew I had a problem.

'After I had the liposuction done, I had to nurse my

dying father and it was a pretty miserable time. I sat around and ate a lot and put on weight. I was really scared that I'd undone the liposuction and that my legs would get fat again – but they didn't.

'They're not racehorse slim by any means. The skin of my thighs was stretched from years of being fat there, so they're not at all firm. But they weren't to start with. And the point is that I feel so much better about them. From time to time I wonder about having more fat removed, but I feel so confident all over now that I'm not sure I'm sufficiently bothered enough to have it done any more.

'My thighs ruled my life, they dictated what I wore, how I spent my time and yes, they made me worried about starting a new relationship when I broke up with a long-standing boyfriend. Anyone who has a hang-up like that should have liposuction.'

Where it works

As the technique of liposuction is refined and improved, the age limit to having it done has been extended to 50 or 55 in cases where it is combined with a tummy tuck or face-lift. It can now be used with varying degrees of success on the following areas:

- beneath the chin, as part of a face-lift in someone older
- on the upper arms, which does not work well
- on the breasts, as part of a breast reduction
- on the abdomen, as part of a tummy tuck
- on the lower back, where the skin is too thick for it to work well

- on the lower part of the abdomen, where it works well if skin is thick
- on the upper part of the abdomen, where it does not work so well
- on the hips (love handles), where it gives excellent results
- on the buttocks, where too much removal of fat creates 'sad' or empty buttocks
- on the outer thigh, where it gives good results
- on the inner thigh, where results are poor because skin is thin
- on the inner part of the knee, which works well
- just above the knee, which doesn't work well
- on the lower leg, where it is less successful but is used around the ankles, though it causes swelling.

Liposuction is frequently marketed as a cure for cellulite. But classical liposuction removes fat at a deeper level than the cellulite (*see page 148*). Removing fat from immediately beneath the skin involves the use of an extremely fine cannula. When combined with fat injections to smooth out bumps, this treatment is called liposculpture. However, liposculpture can cause scarring in the tissues that can show up as irregularities in body shape ten years later, especially after weight loss.

It can be easy to be misled by seductive advertisements from private clinics suggesting that liposuction is a walk-in, walk-out procedure. Although the damage is hidden beneath the skin, it's a major assault on the body that can cause pain and requires time for recovery. There have also been some deaths reported in people who have had liposuction – due to too much fat removed causing severe blood loss.

What is involved

The surgeon should check your general health and advise you to lose excess weight if you need to. You should also be told about the pros and cons of having liposuction.

The operation is normally carried out under general anaesthetic if you are having a large area treated, although a lot of fat – up to 1.5 litres – can safely be removed as a day case. If you have more than that taken out you will need to stay overnight, due to the loss of fluid from your circulation which will have to be replaced. Very occasionally when a large amount of fat is being removed, a blood transfusion is necessary.

Before the operation, you will have the areas to be treated marked out by the surgeon and then you will be put to sleep. Fat is removed either by a dry technique or a wet (tumescent) technique, where the area to be treated will be injected with a mixture of saline, local anaesthetic (which lasts eight hours), adrenaline (to stop bleeding) and a drug called hyalase to allow this fluid to penetrate the body fat. Roughly, the same amount of fluid is injected as the amount of fat to be sucked out.

The surgeon takes a fine cannula (just 3mm in diameter), which comes with different heads and is coupled to a high vacuum chamber, to suck out the fat. Through a small stab wound, the cannula is moved in different directions to suck out enough fat from that particular area, then moved to another. The surgeon will keep feeling the skin to check that fat is being removed evenly and that a smooth contour will be left. The surgeon will try to remove as much fat as possible. But some people's fat is more difficult to suck out than other people's.

When one side of the body is finished, the fat will be measured and the same amount removed from the other side.

The fat which is sucked out should be white – not red with blood. It is safest to get down to the deepest layers of fat, although some superficial fat will be taken from places where the surgeon is creating a fold, at the top of the leg, for instance. As much fat as possible will be removed, but there must be some left beneath the skin so it does not stick to muscle.

The amount of time taken to do a liposuction depends on the area treated. For hips and thighs, it will take about an hour. Afterwards a stitch is placed in each incision, wide elastoplast is stuck over treated areas and you will be dressed in an elastic compression garment. This is worn to prevent the accumulation of fluid under the skin and to help skin spring back into shape. When you have recovered from the operation, if you have had only a small amount of fat removed, you can go home. If you have had 2–3 litres removed, you should stay in overnight.

You may feel sore afterwards but you should not be in real pain. Healing is aided by walking around as much as possible. You must keep the pressure garment on for at least three weeks – more if you've had liposuction in the lower leg. The stitches and elastoplast will be removed after ten days.

'I'm extremely tall and had put on a lot of weight while I was working so hard to set up my own business,' says Susanna Stewart, who's 25 and imports oriental giftware. 'And I was about to get married.

> 'So I decided to have liposuction to kick-start myself into starting a diet. The surgeon looked at me and said that he couldn't give me a flat stomach and slim legs, but he

could get rid of the excess fat. However, this was not a quick fix, he warned me. I would have to look after myself.

'I found liposuction incredibly painful. I felt stiff, sore and very bruised for at least two weeks afterwards. But I could see the difference immediately, even though I had to wear elastic compression trousers for two months. I'd got my waist back, my stomach was flatter and my legs were slimmer.

'I was very pleased and felt so much better about myself that I have since lost over 3 st and haven't broken my diet once. However, I wouldn't do it again, because I think it is hard on the body. But I'm really glad to have been helped by liposuction when I needed help.'

The risks

You are unlikely to lose any weight after having liposuction and immediately after the operation the treated area may actually be bigger than it was before. Post-operative swelling means that you will have fluid retention in the treated area that can take three to six months to settle down completely. Some surgeons use drains for the first 24 hours.

The common problems are bruising, the development of haematoma (collections of clotted blood) and seroma (collections of clear fluid), rumpling of skin which is not elastic enough to contract back into shape and numbness (sensation should return in around four to six weeks). Results can be uneven in inexperienced hands. A layer of fat must be left under the skin, if too much is removed, you may be left with a dimpled and ridged skin.

In general, people are very satisfied with liposuction but

occasionally they may be disappointed. Someone with very high expectations may be frustrated by the results as it does take weeks and even months for tissue swelling to go down, so don't jump to the conclusion that it's money down the drain. The end results may take up to six months to show after surgery.

No more than 2–3 litres of fat should be removed at one time because too much blood may be lost. If you have extensive liposuction then you may become anaemic and are advised to take iron supplements for a month. As mentioned, very occasionally, a blood transfusion may be required.

Another unusual side effect is a damaged nerve. This can occur when liposuction is carried out beneath the chin and affects the nerve producing movement of the corner of the mouth. Occasionally there may be persistent fluid retention (oedema), which mainly occurs when liposuction is done on the lower leg.

Liposuction is so popular that there is a lot of money to be made out of it – so it is marketed in as many different guises as possible. And there are several different ways of killing fat cells. Liposuction does it mechanically. It can also be done by using electricity, lasers or ultrasound – high frequency sound waves which break up fat cells like gallstones, turning the fat into oil which is then sucked out.

There is no evidence that any of these methods works better than another, or that one causes less swelling or bruising than another. Some of them take longer to do, but they are all simply different forces to break up the fat.

Cost: around £1,000 to £4,500 depending on the areas treated

Risks: failure of skin to contract; uneven removal of fat; a late risk of liposculpture is irregularity of skin surface

Ideal age: under 35 with good skin tone

Length of stay in hospital: depends on the amount of fat removed

Anaesthetic: general

Other drugs: mild painkillers

Discomfort levels: low

Time before the signs of surgery disappear: three to six months (completely)

Length of time results last: permanent, provided no weight is gained

THE TREATMENT OF CELLULITE

Few of us like the dimpling that occurs in our upper thighs when we cross our legs. However carefully we keep our weight under control and take regular exercise, nothing seems to refine the orange-peel look of that dense stubborn fat.

Many British doctors deny that cellulite is anything other than accumulated fat. But why does it affect normal and even underweight women as well as overweight women?

Cellulite forms at times when hormones are in flux – in puberty, pregnancy, on the Pill and at the menopause – and takes several years to build up. It affects 80 per cent of all Western women, including thin ones. Cellulite may also be found on some men – these men either have unusually high levels of oestrogen or unusually low levels of testosterone.

Female athletes don't get cellulite, so there must be some link with inactivity. People who don't get enough to eat don't get it, so there must be a link with excess food intake. Cellulite also tends to run in families.

There's no strict medical definition of cellulite, which is mainly found on hips and thighs, although it can appear on upper arms, lower legs and on the lower abdomen. However, cosmetic surgeons have been taking more interest in its exact nature.

The primary kind of cellulite forms in the superficial layer of fat which is found immediately below the skin. This layer is made up of regular pockets of dense fat separated by vertical walls of connective tissue. These fibrous side walls are firmly anchored to the under surface of the epidermis (top layer of skin) and to a sheet of membrane covering the deeper layer of fat.

When a person puts on weight and the fat cells expand in this superficial layer, the fibrous walls don't expand, so they pull on the skin causing it to pucker and dimple.

A secondary kind of cellulite may be linked to loss of skin elasticity due to age, sun damage, weight loss or liposuction. This type is found in women aged over 35, whose whole layer of skin and superficial fat has become relaxed and stretched, resulting in droopy soft tissue and cellulite. Unlike the primary kind, secondary cellulite can be helped by having an operation to tighten the skin.

Liposuction is not generally seen as a treatment for cellulite, because it removes much deeper levels of fat, where it is bound more loosely in a haphazard network of partitions. However, Italian surgeons have perfected the use of tiny cannulas to suck out fat closer to the surface of the skin. When combined with fat injections to even out the lumps this treatment is called liposculpture. But, as mentioned, the removal of superficial fat may cause problems in the long term in that, if a woman becomes thinner as she ages, irregularities in her body shape, caused by the liposuction, will begin to show up.

Treatments on offer

Women are so keen to try and get rid of their cellulite that its removal and treatment are big business. There are several different techniques intended to treat cellulite:

Cellulolipolysis. This involves the insertion of eight pairs of fine 6-in needle electrodes into fatty tissue and then switching on an electric current. Treatment is said to alter the electrical charge of fat cells, so they have to expend more energy trying to restore the situation to normal. This causes fat to be burned off. At least six weekly treatments, administered by a nurse under medical instruction, are required.

Mesotherapy. This consists of the injection of various pharmacologically active substances into the fat beneath the skin. Mesotherapy is used by specially trained doctors in parts of Europe – France, Belgium, Spain and Italy, in particular – and Latin America to treat several conditions, including arthritis and neck pain, as well as cellulite. Treatment for cellulite consists of multiple injections over the surface of the leg, once a week. At least five weekly treatments administered by a doctor are said to be required.

Massage and diet. Salon treatments consist basically of

massage, intensified by the use of mitts or bristle brushes, special creams and so-called detoxifying diets. The theory behind detoxification is that you can flush out the toxins which accumulate in cellulite – the body's dustbin. Massage and moisturising cream will temporarily enhance the look of the thighs by plumping up the epidermis and increasing blood flow to the area. Ultrasound is now being used, too, as it is said to break up pockets of fat.

None of these treatments have ever been subjected to a proper clinical trial. If you decide to try one out, you must ask if it is safe, how much it costs, whether you can meet satisfied users and whether you will get your money back if treatment is unsuccessful.

In this shadowy area between beauty therapy and cosmetic surgery, it pays to keep your eyes open.

THE TUMMY TUCK

The tummy tuck operation – or abdominoplasty – removes the loose lax skin and excess fat that affect many women after pregnancy, however many sit-ups and crunches they force themselves to do. Very occasionally, men are candidates for a tummy tuck as well.

The skin and muscles of the outer wall of the abdomen are stretched during pregnancy, which can cause a weakness down the middle of the abdominal muscles or even a hernia – where a section of bowel pokes out through the gap down the middle and shows up as a deformed tummy button sprouting outwards.

Women can suffer real loss of self-esteem because of their so-called prune bellies. They feel inhibited about buying

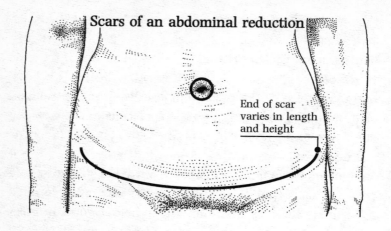

Scars of an abdominal reduction

End of scar
varies in length
and height

clothes, wearing a swimsuit and, of course, in bed.

In the run-up to the menopause, fat starts to be deposited around the waist (rather than on the hips), where it collects beneath loose skin to form rolls of extra flab. Men, too, can also collect this loose extra flab.

However, the tummy tuck operation should not be seen as an alternative to diet and exercise and it should never be undertaken without a serious effort to lose excess fat. Obese people are more likely to develop a deep vein thrombosis in the leg, which may cause a potentially fatal blood clot to travel to the lung.

A stubborn pot belly may be best treated with liposuction, but for people who have an apron of skin hanging down – sometimes made worse by scars from Caesarean delivery, hysterectomy or appendicectomy – the only way to remove it is with surgery, which often includes liposuction.

This operation should only be carried out on people in good health, who have lost excess weight and are fit. Women should not have surgery until they have completed their families. After a tummy tuck, you must avoid gaining weight again.

What is involved

The surgeon will check your general health and weight. He or she will examine your tummy to see that there is enough loose skin to be cut away without stretching the subsequent scar, note any scars that might interfere with healing and see if you have a hernia.

The surgeon will also want to see whether your tummy button can be pulled right down to pubic hair level to check that you have enough loose skin. If you haven't, you may be left with a vertical scar running up to the tummy button, as well as the horizontal one from hip to hip.

The state of your abdominal muscles will also be looked at. If they are weak, you will be told to strengthen them with tummy-toning exercises before you have surgery.

The operation is done under general anaesthetic and requires at least one and possibly two nights in hospital. It entails cutting from hip to hip just above the pubic hair, where there is a natural crease in fatter individuals, and cutting around the tummy button leaving it on a stalk.

The surgeon sucks out any excess fat with liposuction – especially over the hip area – and then frees the skin and fat from the surface of the abdominal muscle. The muscle is tightened and the hernia – if there is one – repaired. Then the skin and fat are drawn downwards, the surplus cut off and the wound stitched up. A new hole is cut out for the tummy button, which is stitched into place. Stitches are all under the skin surface, except around the tummy button, to produce the finest possible scar.

In a modified version of the tummy tuck, called a mini tuck, the tummy button is untouched and simply ends up lower than before when the skin is pulled down.

You will come out of the operating theatre with your knees bent and supported on pillows to take the strain off the scar. Drains will be inserted and removed 24–48 hours later, depending on the amount of fluid. It is very important to get up and move around as soon as possible after the operation. You may be advised to wear a pressure garment for three weeks and stitches are removed after 12 days.

You will be left with a long scar, which should be low enough to be concealed by a bikini, and a small scar around the navel. It will take about a year for the scars to soften and fade.

The risks

The operation causes a lot of soreness. Bruising can prevent your gut from working for 24 hours, so you feel sick and can't eat or drink. Sometimes people find they can't pass urine and have to have a catheter inserted for a while. You're also at risk of a chest infection after surgery.

There is always swelling above the scar where the lymph channels are divided, which may take up to six months to resolve. The wound may become infected, you may develop haematoma (collections of clotted blood) and seroma (collections of clear fluid) and there is always the risk that some of the fat left in your abdomen dies as a result of being interfered with. Occasionally, the straw-coloured fluid in a chronic seroma needs to be drawn off with a syringe.

The scar around the tummy button, which is difficult to disguise, may take a while to heal up. Almost always there will be numbness of the area between the tummy button and pubic hair, caused by damage to a nerve supplying the skin of the abdomen. Very occasionally a patient could be left with numbness and permanent tingling in the front of the thigh, also caused by nerve damage.

'I had an emergency peritonitis operation when I was eight and it left me with a 1-in thick scar running right down the right hand side of my abdomen,' says Judith Cooke, a senior secretary who's 48.

'It sliced my tummy in half and consequently my stomach muscles never worked well. But it never really bothered me until recently. Somehow it wasn't so bad when I was young and attractive. It was only when I was approaching the menopause, that I felt aware of having a disfigured body.

'So I had it rebuilt. I had the damaged muscle repaired by a tummy tuck operation and I had liposuction at the same time. I woke up after the operation feeling some pain, but it wasn't bad. I remember I couldn't turn over in bed or pull myself up. I now have a long thin bikini line scar running from hip to hip – the other was cut away – and a new tummy button and I'm really flat down the front.

'I had the operation at the end of October last year and after a quiet couple of months convalescing, I spent Christmas in the Caribbean. Of course I felt guilty about spending so much money on myself – I paid around £4,500 in all – but the operation was phenomenally successful. I'm so proud of myself now – my self-confidence has been given a huge boost. I'd advise anyone with a disfigurement to have cosmetic surgery. I only wish I'd done it before.'

Cost: around £2,500 (as a day case) and £3,000 (overnight)

Risks: numbness; swelling above scar; poor healing around navel

Ideal age: 40-plus

Length of stay in hospital: one or two nights

Anaesthetic: general

Other drugs: strong painkillers

Discomfort levels: high

Time before the signs of surgery disappear: three to six months

Length of time results last: permanent

CHAPTER NINE

Looking at Limbs

VARICOSE VEINS

Blueish knotted veins bulging out of the leg are unattractive and very common. One in three people is likely to get varicose veins in their lifetime – four to five times as many women as men. Women with varicose veins may hate their legs and be reluctant ever to reveal them.

Surgery is carried out to relieve the tiredness and aching of legs with varicose veins. It is done to prevent the veins from getting worse when there may be long-term complications such as eczema, ulceration of the skin around the ankle and severe bleeding if the leg is injured. It is also done for purely cosmetic reasons.

There are two systems of veins in the legs – a superficial system and a deep one, where blood is pushed back up to the heart. The veins are fitted with one-way valves to stop blood flowing back down again, due to the force of gravity.

When a valve is damaged and fails, blood flows down so that the next valve down the vein is at risk of failure. Blood starts to pool in the veins so the pressure builds up and varicose veins are formed. However, it takes years for them to become severe.

Major damage to the valves can occur either in the groin or in the lower leg. If it occurs in the groin, then surgery is required to remove the major vein (long saphenous vein) through a cut in the groin. This is known as stripping. If damage occurs in the lower leg, the affected veins are disconnected and pulled out through tiny cuts dotted around up the leg, like a bird pulling out a worm. This can sometimes be done under a local anaesthetic.

Pregnant women are particularly vulnerable to varicose veins because of the increased weight and pressure caused by the growing baby, but the tendency is also inherited. Varicose veins are not directly caused by constipation, lack of exercise or the Pill, although pregnancy, obesity and standing for long periods of time are all contributing factors.

If you have to stand for long periods, it's advisable to wear support stockings and avoid clothes which are too tight. Put your feet up but don't cross your legs when sitting. Take regular exercise to boost circulation and try to keep your weight normal.

Surgery should be done as soon as you notice that your legs ache after standing and that you like to put your feet up when you sit down. Women should not wait until after they've completed their family, because the better the veins before pregnancy, the better they will be after it. Removing varicose veins does not increase the stress on remaining veins nor does it cause them to get worse.

What is involved

To do it properly requires very careful analysis of the leg veins before surgery. The surgeon will examine your legs and ideally use an ultrasound machine to assess the state of your veins and build up a road map of the veins in your legs. No one's veins are the same. Ultrasound is a new alternative to x-rays and is the same machine as used to examine a woman's baby when she is pregnant.

When there is a leaking valve in the groin, a general anaesthetic is required. If both legs are operated on you may have to stay in hospital overnight.

After surgery, the leg will be bandaged for the first day or so and it should be raised as much as possible. You will then be advised to wear heavy elastic stockings and encouraged to walk as much as possible. Pain and discomfort are unusual and can be treated with codeine. There may be short-term bruising and swelling. The cuts are so small that they heal very quickly.

'I was 31 when I had my veins done,' says Jessica Collins, who's a fitness instructor now aged 40.

'My first vein appeared when I was 18 and by the time of my operation the back of my left leg looked like an old lady's, lumpy and blue. The leg ached whenever I had to stand still. I was all right running or taking hard exercise, but I hated standing about or gentle strolling.

'I felt no pain after the operation at all – apart from sickness from the general anaesthetic when I woke up. My leg was bandaged right up and I had to keep it dry for a week and walk two miles a day for six weeks, which was fine by me – I was longing to get back to training. I had a 2-in cut hidden in my groin and half a dozen tiny cuts in my calf and thigh which all soon faded.

'I was pleased with the results and happy to wear shorts again for several years. But, nearly ten years on, the veins are back, even though I've done everything I can to look after my legs – including lots of exercise and eating healthily. It's my job to be healthy, after all. And I

haven't even had children. So I've booked another operation for a few weeks' time.'

The risks

The commonest complication is that all the affected veins
are often not dealt with and that is why the veins come
back. Many operations are secondary surgery that might
not have been necessary if the first operation was complete.

Some patients are unhappy with the little scars on their
legs left by the stab incisions during surgery. Very occasionally, the operation may cause damage to the superficial
nerves of the leg, leaving areas of numbness in the foot or
upper thigh.

Six weeks after surgery, the patient will be asked to come
and see the surgeon, who will look at the legs and inject any
little blue veins left behind. This treatment is called sclerotherapy and it is often used when surgery is not required. An
irritant solution is injected into the vein, causing the walls to
stick together and the vein eventually to disappear – a
process that takes a few weeks. However, if this irritant fluid
leaks out, it will cause dark brown patches and hardening.

Another common condition linked with varicose veins is
the development of patches of red or blue spider veins (*see
page 99*) on the mid thighs. These little broken capillaries can
often show up on the legs of women in their thirties and may
be a sign of high pressure in the venous system, which will
mean that varicose veins may be developing inside, if they
have not already done so. The spider veins can be treated
with microsclerotherapy, which can leave marks if injected
outside the capillary, or lasers. Spider veins have a tendency
to recur and treatment is not 100 per cent successful.

Cost: surgery can be done on the NHS in some cases. However, there is a huge number of people with varicose veins and only a small number of busy surgeons. Privately, a package deal costs from around £1,700 to £2,350, depending on the extent of surgery

Risks: incomplete surgery

Ideal age: whenever symptoms occur

Length of stay in hospital: one night maximum

Anaesthetic: general, occasionally local

Other drugs: none

Discomfort levels: low

Time before the signs of surgery disappear: a week

Length of time results last: should be permanent, if surgery is complete

THE THIGH-LIFT

A thigh-lift is not recommended for someone who simply has fat thighs. It is an operation that is most often carried out on people who have been very obese and have lost a lot of weight, leaving folds of empty skin where the fat used to be.

It is also sometimes performed on people who have had liposuction on the inner thighs. The skin in this area is very thin and has poor tone, especially if it has been stretched over a vast expanse of fat for several years, so when fat is removed it leaves empty folds of skin. There are three types of thigh-lift. In the first one, the surgeon cuts into the thigh and removes as much fat as is safe and then sews up the cut, which runs in the inside of the groin from the front of the thigh, between the legs and round into the crease beneath the buttocks, where they meet the thighs.

The second type of operation is carried out on more extreme cases where people have excess skin running right the way down to the knee. In these cases, the surgeon will make the same cut in the groin and a second cut running vertically down the inside of the thigh to the knee, which will leave a noticeable scar.

The third type of operation is for people who have been left with 'sad' empty buttocks after weightloss. This 'bottom-lift' involves a cut in the crease below the buttocks which runs all the way round and up to the hip bone.

In the first and third type of operation, the scar is concealed by a fold of flesh. But with the passing of the years, as skin becomes looser and droops downwards, these scars will start to show. This is the major problem with thigh-lifts. They are major operations which cause long scars. You will be immobilised for three or four days. Catheterisation of the bladder is usually required and you may become constipated. You will also have to wear a pressure garment.

Scars can easily become infected. And the risks of fat dying off and the development of seroma (collections of clear fluid) are higher than usual. Nerves are sometimes cut leaving areas of numbness and there may be swelling of the thighs and the lower legs. Sometimes patients complain that the scar on the inner thighs pulls on the labia (vaginal lips).

In people who have lost vast amounts of weight, a thigh-lift is occasionally combined with a tummy tuck and the removal of fat from the hips and buttocks. This huge operation leaves a massive scar.

Cost: around £5,000

Risks: infection; noticeable scars; numbness; swelling

Ideal age: anyone who has lost a lot of weight

Length of stay in hospital: three to four days

Anaesthetic: general

Other drugs: antibiotics

Time before the signs of surgery disappear: six months but scars will be permanent

Length of time results last: permanent

ARM REDUCTION

Hate going sleeveless because of wobbly upper arms? No matter how well-toned your triceps – the muscles at the back of the upper arm – excess skin and fat still gather in this area once you're over 30. Women who have gained and lost weight repeatedly, a cycle which causes the skin to lose its elasticity, are particularly prone to these 'bat wings'. Some women develop such large upper arms that they can't fit into shop-bought clothes.

Liposuction is not an ideal treatment for bat wings because it leaves a floppy empty bag of skin that may look even worse than wobbly fat, but you can have surgery to reduce the upper arm. The problem with an arm reduction is that it leaves a visible scar, because the surgeon cuts down the length of the inside upper arm, from armpit to elbow, to remove a lemon slice of skin and fat.

Most surgeons would advise against an arm reduction except in extreme situations.

Cost: £1,500–£2,000

Risks: noticeable scar

Ideal age: any age

Length of stay in hospital: day case

Anaesthetic: general

Other drugs: none

Discomfort levels: moderate

Time before the signs of surgery disappear: three to six months but scars are permanent

Length of time results last: permanent

THE HANDS

Hands are the true giveaway of your age, unlike the face, which can be modified by many of the treatments outlined earlier. Many forms of treatment are advocated for the wrinkled skin and gaunt look of older hands, including peeling, fat injections, Retin A, collagen injections and even excising excess skin.

Overall, these treatments are disappointing and not widely practised by reputable surgeons in the UK.

CALF AUGMENTATION

Legs can be made more shapely with silicone implants to plump out narrow calves. Women who feel their lower legs are too thin for them to look attractive wearing skirts, sportsmen with spindly shanks and bodybuilders who can't

bulk out their calves may all benefit from calf augmentation. But the people who usually seek this operation are
people who have suffered from paralysis, such as polio,
leaving one or both legs underdeveloped.

The surgeon will examine your legs. Sometimes legs are
shapeless because of fat distribution around and above the
ankles. These legs might be improved with liposuction to
remove the fat rather than calf implants.

Implants are made of hard silicone, which has the consistency of a rubber eraser. They are usually around 5–6in
long and $1^1/_2$–2in wide, although specially tailored implants
can be made.

The operation is carried out under general anaesthetic
with you lying on your front. The implant is inserted through
a small opening in the back of the knee and a pocket is
created to accommodate it on the inner side of the calf, below
the existing muscle. In cases where the leg is very wasted,
two implants may be required, on both the inner and outer
side of the calf.

It is very important that the surgeon does not make the
pocket too big because the implant must stay in position – as
deep as possible below the muscle, to avoid hardening
around the implant. This can occur as a result of internal
scarring which contracts around the implant, causing the
edge of the implant to curl which could spoil the look of the
leg. Other risks include nerve damage causing numbness,
the development of seroma (collections of clear fluid) and
asymmetry because the implant has moved or was put in
wrong.

Calf augmentation is an easy operation for the surgeon to
do, but it can take a while for the implant to settle down. The
leg may be swollen and uncomfortable for the first two days

and you may be advised to stay in hospital for two nights. Once you have recovered from the operation, you may move around as much as you like. But it may take about eight weeks before your legs feel comfortable.

Cost: around £3,000

Risks: hardening of the implant

Ideal age: any age

Length of stay in hospital: two nights maximum

Anaesthetic: general

Other drugs: painkillers

Discomfort levels: medium to high

Time before the signs of surgery disappear: a week

Length of time results last: permanent

CHAPTER TEN

Cosmetic Surgery for Men

PENIS AUGMENTATION

Many men feel that their penises are simply not big enough, although in fact very few are technically underendowed.

In the United States, research – carried out when several unhappy men started complaining of miserable complications such as impotence, after undergoing surgery to lengthen their penises – revealed that the average male erection is just over 5in (12.8cm).

This figure is just an average, which means there are many men who have 4-in erections and many who have 7-in erections. Men do vary enormously in size.

But just over 5in is shorter than popularly assumed and may help men come to terms with what they've got, rather than opting for a risky operation. Most men tend to worry more about the length of their penis in its normal state – that is, when it isn't erect. But very few men truly suffer from what doctors call micropenis – short penis – which can occur when there is not enough of the male hormone, testosterone, in the body.

A Chinese surgeon called Dr Long was the first to popularise the operation to lengthen the penis. He and his colleagues located the suspensory ligament that lies between the pubic bone and the top of the genitals and holds the erect penis close to the abdomen. When it is cut, the length of penis that lies inside the pubic bone drops forward and is exposed.

The ligament is then divided and reattached lower down on the pubic bone so that the penis is extended by around 20 per cent to 50 per cent, depending on which surgeon you believe. The skin can stretch to accommodate the new length. Side effects include an erection that starts rather lower down, sticks straight out rather than up and may be a bit wobbly. There may also be pubic hair on top of the shaft, which may require shaving. The scar in the pubic region is hidden by hair.

Men who desire width rather than length may decide to have fat injected into their penises.

About 3oz of fat may be liposuctioned out of the tummy wall and washed before being injected into the base of the artificially erect penis. About 40 per cent of this fat is expected to remain but the rest will be absorbed. The operation can be repeated after six months. Fat injections make the penis thicker – until the fat is eventually absorbed – but leave the size of the glans unchanged. The problem with fat injections is that results are unpredictable. If some of the fat survives and there is scarring, it may result in a knobbly surface. So surgeons have tended to carry out dermal fat grafts, where a strip of skin (with the surface layer removed) is slipped under the skin of the penis through a cut and wrapped around its length like a scarf.

If you choose to have anything done to your penis, you will have to refrain from penetrative sex for at least six weeks afterwards and the recovery time is usually longer, with pain, bleeding and swelling.

Results are thought to be pretty unsatisfactory. Surgery can lead to loss of sensation, infection leading to skin problems and deformity, which in turn can lead to such severe psychological distress that no erection will be possible at all.

Surgery is rarely advisable for the group of anxious men who have a normal-sized organ but fear they aren't big enough. It's quite likely that these men have a psychosexual problem. Men should be reassured by their partners that it's what they do with their penis that matters – not its size.

Cost: lengthening, around £4,000; widening, around £750

Risks: variable swelling; infection leading to scarring; contour deformity; major functional problems

Ideal age: any

Length of stay in hospital: none

Anaesthetic: general (day case)

Other drugs: painkillers, antibiotics

Discomfort levels: high

Time before the signs of surgery disappear: two months

Length of time results last: not known

BREAST REDUCTION

Many men are unhappy about having protruding breasts that no amount of diet or exercise will shift. This condition is called gynaecomastia and it is surprisingly common. In fact weight lifters who take steroids to build up their pectoral muscles can often find they develop breast tissue behind the nipples. This is because gynaecomastia can be a side effect of taking any of 40 to 50 medicinal drugs, including steroids and oestrogens.

However, the condition usually develops in puberty, when around one in three boys will have some degree of gynaecomastia, sometimes in one breast, sometimes in two. With time, the breasts usually go down again to the boy's satisfaction and reassurance is all that is needed.

But some adolescents and adult men – who are sometimes overweight – have larger breasts which can be a source of great psychological distress. For these men, surgery can help. And it is becoming increasingly popular. In the US, the number of men who had surgery to reduce their breasts doubled from 5,000 in 1992 to 10,000 in 1994.

The surgeon will want a medical drug history and will make a full medical examination to ensure that development is normal. He or she will examine your breasts to find out whether they are made of glandular tissue or fat.

Fatty breasts: if breasts only consist of fat, then it can be removed by liposuction (*see page 139*), with incisions being made either in the areola (the coloured part around the nipple) or in the armpit. A compression vest must be worn for a month after surgery to ensure that the skin contracts properly.

Glandular breasts: if the breasts are made up of glandular tissue, then it will have to be cut out. A small incision is made in the shape of a C, halfway round the areola and the nipple is lifted up on a bed of tissue. Leaving this pad of glandular tissue should ensure that when the rest of it is removed, the breast is not left completely flat.

The operation is done as a day case under general anaesthetic. Drains will be inserted and it will take ten days or so for your chest to recover. The scar usually heals well, but there will be bruising for three to four weeks.

The main risk is that too much tissue and/or fat will be removed, leaving a flat-looking chest. If your breasts were very large and the skin does not contract, then you will be left with an empty pouch that still makes you look as though you've got breasts. This skin can be removed by the surgeon but you will be left with very noticeable scars. There may also be irregular healing inside, so that your breasts ruckle up afterwards. In addition, there may be loss of sensation in the nipple. There is always the possible complication of developing haematoma (collections of clotted blood), but they should resolve on their own, although they may require removal.

Cost: £2,000–£2,500

Risks: flat chest; empty bags or haematoma

Ideal age: any age over 18

Length of stay in hospital: none

Anaesthetic: general (day case)

Other drugs: strong painkillers

Discomfort levels: medium to high

Time before the signs of surgery disappear: three months or more

Length of time results last: permanent

PECTORAL AUGMENTATION

Pectoral implants may be desired by bodybuilders wanting to add the finishing touches to their physique. It's fashionable on the West Coast of America but still rarely asked for in the UK. But individually tailored solid silicone implants are most often used to treat men with an undeveloped, lopsided or sunken chest.

Implants are inserted through a small incision in the armpit, where hair will conceal the scar. Implants can be from 1–5cm thick. They are placed as deep as possible beneath the pectoral muscles throwing muscle bulk forward. The deeper the implant is placed, the less risk there is of scar tissue contracting around the implant, causing hardening.

The most common problem is that the body may react against the foreign objects by producing a lot of fluid (seroma), which must be drained off. It is important not to move the drains too early otherwise the chest may blow up with fluid which will then have to be sucked out. Most patients can go home the day after surgery with the drains still in if there is excess fluid production. Otherwise there is always a small risk of infection after surgery. But this operation is usually fairly straightforward.

Cost: £2,500–£3,500

Risks: excess fluid

Ideal age: any age

Length of stay in hospital: one to two nights

Anaesthetic: general

Other drugs: antibiotics if necessary

Discomfort levels: high

Time before the signs of surgery disappear: scar is hidden in armpit

Length of time results last: permanent

ABDOMINAL ETCHING

Men who pump iron can find it hard to show off their abdominal muscles, because the 'abs' don't show unless a lot of fat is lost, which can mean losing muscle mass as well. A new technique available in the United States, called abdominal etching, uses liposuction to remove a tablespoon of fat from the central crease of the abdominal muscle upwards from the tummy button. Fat can also be removed from along the edges of the muscle. A general anaesthetic is required, even though only a small amount of fat is removed. This procedure for men is simply a further use of liposuction.

LIPOINFILTRATION

Another new cosmetic technique being tried out in the United States is lipoinfiltration. This is a method of beefing up pectoral muscles, biceps and even calves by transplanting fat into the muscle. The aim is to extract fat from the abdomen by syringe and then place it as deep into the muscle as possible, through an incision rather than by injecting it. This technique is said to be less damaging to fat cells and it is claimed that the deeply embedded fat is not absorbed. There is no good evidence that having fat injected anywhere in the body actually works and there is a risk with this procedure of scarring in the muscle.

CHAPTER ELEVEN

Genital Surgery for Women

Genital surgery can be technically simple for the surgeon to carry out. But the surgeon will want to be completely sure that anyone who seeks such surgery has a genuine cause for concern. We are all slightly different and the sexual parts of our bodies can cause us great anxiety. So if you seek surgery, do not take it amiss if the surgeon refers you to a counsellor or sex therapist for an evaluation, which may include a physical examination.

Here are some of the more common procedures which surgeons carry out.

VAGINAL REDUCTION

A number of women request surgery to reduce their enlarged vaginas. An oversized and stretched vagina reduces sexual sensation for both partners and a vaginal reduction, when it is necessary, can bring about a great improvement.

The usual reason for an enlarged vagina is childbirth. But older, post-menopausal women can find their vaginas have enlarged, too, and those who have been treated for cervical cancer sometimes feel the need to seek vaginal reconstruction.

However, some women may mistakenly believe that their vaginas are too large as a result of hurtful comments by thoughtless partners. This is when reassurance is necessary, not surgery.

At your first consultation, the surgeon will take your medical history and examine you internally to make sure that your vagina really is too big. If the surgeon is male, you might like to bring along a friend or partner to act as chaperone, or ask for a secretary or receptionist to be present in the room. This can reassure you and protect the surgeon from allegations of indecency.

The aim of the operation is to recreate a narrow vagina. You will be given a general anaesthetic and will most likely stay in hospital overnight. The surgeon will remove a wedge-shaped section of vaginal wall from the back, where the vagina is separated from the anus by the perineum – the elastic fan-shaped tissue that is stretched and sometimes cut or torn during childbirth. Muscle and skin are rejoined with stitches.

Any discomfort afterwards is similar to that of an episiotomy – where the perineum is cut during childbirth – which can be very painful. But the area usually heals well and should feel fine in about ten days, although you may feel nervous about engaging in penetrative sex for a while longer.

A common problem is that the surgeon may overtighten the vagina, so that penetrative sex is uncomfortable. But the scar soon stretches and the problem quickly resolves.

Cost: around £2,000

Risks: none

Ideal age: any, after completing a family

Length of stay in hospital: one night

Anaesthetic: general

Other drugs: moderate painkillers and antibiotics

Discomfort levels: medium

Time before the signs of surgery disappear: up to three weeks or so

Length of time results last: permanent

LABIAL SURGERY

It is not unusual for a woman to be dissatisfied with her labia minora – the inner lips of the vagina. Everyone is constructed slightly differently and women's genitalia are more or less hidden. However, larger than average cauliflower labia may protrude well beyond the outer lips of the vagina and cause discomfort when they rub against clothing or during sex.

It is possible for a surgeon to trim the labia if they are larger than average. But first you will need to be examined to make sure that surgery is necessary – some women may mistakenly believe that their genitalia are somehow 'wrong', as a result of hurtful comments by a thoughtless partner. You may want to bring a friend or partner or ask a chaperone to be present during this examination.

The operation is usually carried out as a day case under general anaesthetic. But it can be done under a local anaesthetic and the surgeon may suggest using an epidural block, normally used as pain relief in childbirth. An epidural is an anaesthetic, given by injection into the lower spine, which causes numbness from the waist down. It will allow you to remain conscious during the operation so you can instruct the surgeon as to exactly how you want your labia to look. They can then be trimmed according to your wishes and then stitched over the edges so that they heal well.

It is very important that such a sensitive spot should heal well so there is no possibility of painful sex afterwards. In fact, there are usually no post-operative complications.

Cost: £500 (local) – £1,500 (general – day case)

Risks: that reduction does not meet your expectations

Ideal age: 20-plus

Length of stay in hospital: none

Anaesthetic: general or local epidural

Other drugs: mild painkillers

Discomfort levels: medium

Time before the signs of surgery disappear: within a month

Length of time results last: permanent

HYMEN REINSTATEMENT

Women who come from countries where virginity is highly prized sometimes seek surgery to reinstate their hymens before going home to be married. They have to appear to be virginal.

The aim of surgery is to rejoin the remnants of the hymen. It is a straightforward operation which is carried out under general anaesthetic and can be done as a day case, since there should be no pain afterwards nor any complications.

The surgeon stitches the hymen back together with a

dozen or so dissolvable stitches, leaving a small hole for menstruation. Another way of achieving the same effect is by tightening up the back rim of the vagina with a few dissolvable stitches, to create a much narrower orifice.

Whichever way it is done, when penetrative sex next takes place, tissue will be torn and blood will spill on to the marital sheets.

Cost: £1,500

Risks: none

Ideal age: any

Length of stay in hospital: none

Anaesthetic: general

Other drugs: none

Discomfort levels: low

Time before the signs of surgery disappear: a week

Length of time results last: until penetrative sex takes place

CHAPTER TWELVE

Teeth

A sparkling smile lights up a face in a flash but it can be ruined just as quickly if a mouthful of chipped, crowded, protruding, dirty-looking and absent teeth are revealed. Cosmetic dentistry can help you achieve an attractive set of shining teeth.

There has been a growing interest in cosmetic dentistry as more and more people are hanging on to their teeth. Most dental decay occurs before the age of 25, and after that it's a case of maintenance and repair work as fillings degenerate.

High-tech dentistry can save teeth and bridge gaps so successfully that false teeth should soon become a thing of the past. But teeth still show signs of age. They tend to yellow and become more brittle, so they chip and fracture, and they wear down, so they look less sharp and pointed.

More of a worry, in health terms, is creeping gum disease, caused by the build-up of plaque, which affects most of us as we get older and, unchecked, causes teeth to fall out.

Daily brushing and flossing are vital to remove plaque and so are regular visits to the dentist for descaling, when you can ask about improving the look of your teeth.

Today a dentist can straighten them out, fill gaps, conceal chips and improve their colour. Sometimes there are several ways in which faults can be improved, so always ask for alternatives. Some techniques are considerably more expensive than others.

The dentist should always investigate the entire mouth area before recommending a particular course of action. Routine repair dentistry may sometimes have to be carried out before cosmetic work, which should never be done to disguise deeper dental problems.

However, nothing the dentist does for your teeth will last for ever. There are no guarantees when it comes to dental work. Teeth do a lot of hard work every day.

STRAIGHTENING TEETH

We're used to seeing children with a mouthful of wire, but there's no age limit to orthodontic work (teeth straightening). You can have it done in your seventies. Results are simply slower in old age, when it takes longer to move teeth around in the mouth to straighten them out.

Any dentist may carry out orthodontic treatment, but specialists (orthodontists) are more highly qualified. The dentist or orthodontist will look at your teeth, take x-rays and make plaster models of both jaws. If a jaw is overcrowded, it may be necessary to extract some teeth to make room for the others before active treatment begins. Sometimes orthodontic treatment is combined with surgery to correct the position of the jaws.

Crooked teeth are straightened by wearing a personally tailored brace – a fixed or movable device that fits around the teeth and pulls and pushes them into line. Fixed appliances are temporarily bonded to the teeth and they can be made of ceramic or even plastic, so they are less visible. Proper cleaning of the teeth is essential while they are being treated, to prevent decay. Whatever is done to one or two teeth affects the whole set, upper and lower, which must produce a comfortable bite.

When treatment is finished it may be necessary to continue wearing a retainer at night to hold the teeth in their new position. The whole process can at times cause considerable discomfort and aching. Treatment may take up to two years. It requires frequent visits to the orthodontist – about every four to six weeks. But it can transform a jumble into a neat line. Hollywood perfection is not always possible but results can be excellent.

No permanent guarantee can be given, because teeth tend to shift around a little throughout our lives, but it is unlikely that you will need any further treatment.

'I was 27 when I decided to get my teeth fixed,' says Julie Piper, a social worker who's now 33.

> 'I'd always been embarrassed by their crookedness and used to hold my hand up to hide my mouth whenever I smiled. Also, once my wisdom teeth had come through, they made one of the bottom front teeth move right inwards, so my tongue kept hitting it and getting ulcers.
>
> 'I had already had two teeth out when I was eleven and had been fitted with a removable brace, but I never wore it because I found it difficult to talk with it in.
>
> 'This time, I was referred by my dentist to an ortho-dontist at an NHS hospital, who removed two more teeth – the molars next to the eye teeth – under local anaesthetic. Then I was fitted with permanent braces. I wore the top one for just over a year and the bottom one for 18 months.
>
> 'I found it difficult to eat and painful to talk at first. I had to put wax on the fittings to stop them scraping the inside

of my mouth every time I moved it. And every time the braces were tightened up it was excruciatingly painful for a few days. But I never minded how I looked with them. One man even said he found braces sexy, and they do seem to be fashion accessories now.

'Still, it was nice when they were removed and I could see how straight my teeth had become. I had to wear a retainer at night, but even so, my bottom teeth started to move back into their old position. So this time, my orthodontist cut the gums holding the teeth in position, under a local anaesthetic, and I had a brace fixed for another six months. He said if my teeth moved again, there would be nothing he could do. So far they've been fine and I get a lot of compliments now.'

Cost: Some orthodontic work is available free on the NHS for children under 18 and students under 19. For adults, the NHS charge is 80 per cent of the NHS cost, up to £300. This charge is altered from time to time. However, many dentists will only do orthodontic work privately, when costs can easily reach £1,500 and more

DENTAL CONTOURING

Another technique to improve crooked teeth consists of planing away any obviously protruding angles and filing down over-long or pointed teeth to create a smoother look. This is called dental contouring.

Cost: around £25 a tooth

TOOTH WHITENING

Teeth are sometimes discoloured as a result of a knock to them in childhood, before the adult teeth were properly formed. But the big culprits when it comes to staining are tea, coffee and tobacco.

Your dentist will be able to tell you whether staining is on the inside or outside of your teeth. If the nerve of a tooth dies, then discoloration can develop in the pulp cavity inside the tooth. This is treatable with hydrogen peroxide to bleach the inside of the dead tooth. The tooth is drilled open, a bleach-soaked cotton wool ball is inserted and the tooth is temporarily sealed for a week.

Stains on the surface of the teeth can often be polished away by a dental hygienist with microbrasion, which works like sand-blasting and can root out many stubborn stains. If a tooth can't be cleaned up because it has a poor surface caused by defective enamel, then you're best off with a veneer (*see page 184*). Bleaching the outside of the tooth is not allowed in Britain or Europe. This is because tooth whiteners containing more than a tiny amount of hydrogen peroxide (or carbamide peroxide) are currently banned by an EC Directive on safety grounds.

The British Dental Association is concerned that people are being denied an effective treatment for certain types of tooth discoloration and is urging that the ban be lifted. There is also concern about whitening products which can be purchased for use at home. Little information is available about how safe or effective these products are or even what their ingredients are, so the British Dental Association cannot endorse their use.

Cost: £6.64 for a scale and polish under the NHS, £40 to £60 privately; internal bleaching, £150–£250

VENEERS

A veneer is a wafer-thin shell usually made of porcelain that is bonded to the surface of a tooth to improve its appearance. Veneers are the easiest way to achieve perfect-looking white teeth. They can hide a multitude of sins and they last well, resisting chips, cracks and stains.

The dentist will take an impression of the tooth using a putty-like material and this mould is sent to a dental technician together with a colour match – teeth come in a wide range of whites.

When your custom-made veneer is ready, the dentist paints a conditioner on to the tooth to roughen its surface and then a plastic resin with the porcelain veneer on top. This is bonded to the tooth with ultraviolet light.

Advances in dentistry mean that it is now possible for resins to be bonded directly to the live layer of dentine beneath the surface enamel of the tooth. This is helpful for people who have advanced gum disease, where the dentine is exposed at the margin of the gum.

Cost: £53 per tooth under the NHS, between £100 and £450 privately

COSMETIC BONDING

Chipped irregular teeth can be improved by cosmetic bonding, where white filling material is bonded to the tooth and then polished. Made of plastic and finely ground minerals, the white filling material can also be used to build up teeth and close unsightly gaps between them.

However, some dentists prefer to fit veneers because bonding rarely lasts for longer than two to five years. It chips and stains, particularly round the edges. So if you want to keep it white, you will have to cut right down on tea, coffee and cigarettes.

Cost: From £60 to £90 a tooth

CROWNS AND CAPS

Still the best way of disguising heavily filled or broken teeth, crowns and caps are false covers fitted over a tooth which has been drilled down to a cone shape. The strongest crowns are made of gold with a porcelain veneer.

The tooth is prepared at one visit and a mould sent to the dental laboratory, where a technician makes a crown to match. At the second appointment, the crown is filled with dental cement and pushed down over the stump of the original tooth. A light anaesthetic may be used, but the procedure should not hurt.

The crown can last for years – some are bonded to metal for extra strength – but it will not protect the underlying tooth from decay. Bridgework consists of preparing adjacent teeth and putting a crown right across using bonding material.

Cost: £300–£500 depending on materials used

IMPLANTS

Until recently the only options for missing teeth were dentures or bridge work. A denture entails wearing a plastic plate in the mouth and a bridge involves the preparation of adjacent teeth in order to attach a crown right across the gap, using bonding material. But now you can have implants – false teeth anchored to the bone, which will work and look exactly like the real things.

Implants are fitted in three stages. Surgery is required to insert the metal stud (made of pure titanium) into the jaw bone. This is done under a local or general anaesthetic and there will be some discomfort afterwards, due to stitches in the gum which have to stay in place for seven to ten days.

The bone then fuses around the stud in a process called osseointegration, which actually strengthens the jaw. This takes three months for the lower jaw, six months for the top one. When the jaw is ready, a titanium post is screwed into the stud. This post sticks out of the gum, but it can be concealed for a week or so by a temporary bridge. Finally, a permanent false tooth is fixed to it.

You do not need an implant for each missing tooth. Five or six implants can support ten to 12 teeth.

Commitment is required for this lengthy process, which must be carried out by an expert, but results are extremely good, particularly in the lower jaw. Current implants have a success rate of more than 90 per cent in the lower jaw over a 15-year period. However, they are expensive.

Cost: Around £1,200 to £2,000 per tooth

RECEDING GUMS

Gums recede and deteriorate with age, but dentists have made moderate progress in transferring gum tissue from one location to another, although they will never look the same as they did in youth. Gums can also be cut away if they are too obtrusive. Gum surgery is sometimes done with a laser, although this is still in its infancy.

HOW TO FIND A COSMETIC DENTIST

You can always ask your dentist to refer you to a specialist in the kind of cosmetic dental work you are wanting, or you can look up names in your local edition of *Yellow Pages*. But the usual route is personal recommendation – people tend to ask their friends.

You may have to shop around for the right dentist or orthodontist for your requirements. If you pass a dental surgery, pop in and make some inquiries about the kind of work they do.

You can always ring the General Dental Council (tel: 0171 486 2171) and ask about a particular dentist's qualifications. But neither the General Dental Council nor the British Dental Association can recommend names.

All dentists will have the letters BDS (Bachelor of Dental Surgery) and/or LDSRCS (Licentiate Dental Surgeon of the Royal College of Surgeons) after their name and there is a huge range of other qualifications.

Dentists who have had further training in orthodontics may have any of the following letters after their names – D Orth (Diploma in Orthodontics), M Orth (Membership in Orthodontics), MDO (Membership in Dental Orthodontics), DD Orth (Diploma in Dental Orthodontics) and FDS (Fellowship in Dental Surgery). And an MSc (Master of Science) could also be in orthodontics.

None of these qualifications necessarily mean that the

dentist regularly practises as an orthodontist and some have none of these letters after their names, because the qualifications did not exist when they were in training.

CHAPTER THIRTEEN

Covering Up Baldness

All mammals have hair. We have it on our heads to keep us warm because we lose so much heat through our scalp. Each hair is produced by a follicle under the skin and spends around three years growing and three months resting before falling out. At any one time around 90 per cent of the hairs on our head are growing and 10 per cent are resting. We lose around 100 hairs a day.

There are two types of hair – vellous hair, which is fine, soft, baby hair and terminal hair. Vellous hair can change into terminal hair, as it does when an adolescent needs to start shaving, and terminal hair can change into vellous hair, as it does when a man is balding.

Our hair pattern is determined by the number of terminal hairs we have on our head and this is affected by our genes and by our health and emotional wellbeing. Women have more hair than men. During pregnancy it becomes more plentiful and it falls out during breastfeeding.

The most common cause of permanent hair loss is male pattern baldness or androgenic alopecia. Eunuchs do not suffer baldness, as the ancient Greek physician, Hippocrates, noted. Throughout the ages, men have sought a cure for their baldness. The oldest known medical text includes a home remedy consisting of the fat of a lion, a hippopotamus, a crocodile, a serpent and an ibex.

More recently, doctors have tried treating baldness with injections of the female sex hormone. High doses of oestrogen will arrest the progression of baldness and may cause hair to grow, but the side effects amount to castration – including loss of sex drive, breast enlargement and changes in the distribution of body hair.

With the passing of the years, some baldness will affect 65 per cent of men. It can begin as early as the age of 18 and be established by 35. A man cannot predict how he will look from the appearance of his father since male pattern baldness, which is genetically determined, is passed down the female line.

Causes of hair loss

Loss of hair in men is triggered by production of the androgen hormone, which starts to decline in the late twenties. So if a man still has a full head of hair by the time he is 45, he is likely to keep it.

Long-term stress and an unhealthy lifestyle may contribute to earlier and faster balding in men. When the body is under stress it pours out adrenaline in the fight-or-flight response. This triggers the release of more androgen, so promoting balding.

Women with thinning hair may also be producing more androgen as a result of stress. There is often a thinning of the hair after the menopause. This is partly due to the decline in oestrogen which means that the ratio of circulating androgen goes up, triggering a fall in the number of active follicles on the scalp. It's also due to a slowing down in the rate of hair growth and to hair becoming drier and finer in texture.

This process starts before the menopause, but it may not be noticed until a woman is in her fifties because we can lose a lot of hair from our heads before it looks sparse. Men can lose up to half their hair before we describe them as balding. In old age many men and women display the thin wispy tendrils of baby vellous hair.

Does nutrition have anything to do with a healthy head of hair? A poor diet forces the body to conserve essential nutrients for vital organs, rather than hair (or nails). Thinning hair can be connected with a deficiency of the minerals iron, zinc and copper and the thickness and lustre of animal fur is improved by the B vitamins (brewers' yeast is a good source). Otherwise, it's simply a question of eating well.

In the future, there'll doubtless come a day when we'll be able to have hair follicles cultured in a test tube and implanted in the scalp by the thousands. Even better, there'll be gene therapy to stop hair dropping out in the first place. Or there'll be effective anti-androgens that suppress the male hormones while avoiding feminisation.

Pharmaceutical companies stand to make millions from an effective anti-balding product. But to date just one drug, apart from hormones, has any effect at all. Minoxidil is a drug which widens blood vessels and is used to treat raised blood pressure. It has the curious side effect of encouraging hair growth.

Painting a weak solution of minoxidil (not strong enough to have any effect on blood pressure) on the scalp twice a day may reduce hair loss and promote some fine regrowth – which falls out when the treatment is stopped – after six months. But results satisfy only about one in ten men. In US tests, 41 per cent of women using minoxidil for eight months showed no regrowth at all and of those who did 40 per cent had only minimal regrowth.

Another drug is in the pipeline. Proscar is an anti-androgen drug that has been approved in the US as treatment for an enlarged prostate. It does not cause feminisation because it does not act on all androgens, just the ones that cause baldness. Results have yet to be proved, but Proscar may work for women with hair loss too.

All we really have at present for the man who can't accept his hairless destiny is improvements in hair replacement surgery and advances in hair-weaving. Put yourself in the hands of an expert and you really can have your baldness permanently concealed.

The only trouble is that it's extremely difficult to find an expert. Most of the good surgeons – that is, the ones who are skilled at hair replacement surgery – are in the United States, South America, France and Scandinavia, but not particularly in Britain.

So what can a top surgeon offer you?

PUNCH GRAFTS (MICROGRAFTS)

The basic principle of all hair replacement surgery is simply to move hair from an area where it is genetically programmed to remain thick – the back and sides – to areas where it will fall out – the temples and crown.

A punch graft is a small circular plug of skin and underlying fat some 4–5mm in diameter containing 10 to 20 hairs. It is removed from the back and sides of the hair (the resulting hole is closed with a stitch) and inserted into a small incision prepared in the balding area.

The major drawback of a punch graft is that a dappled effect is created in the back and sides of the hair where they have been removed and a toothbrush effect is created where they are transplanted – the visible tufts giving the artificial appearance of a doll's head.

Today, the technique has been refined and an expert surgeon will take a strip of hair-bearing skin from the back of the head, sew up the split and divide the 10-cm long graft into tiny plugs containing just two or three hairs apiece. These micrografts are then inserted into pinholes created by a laser, making sure that they are put in at the correct angle so the hair grows the right way.

What is involved

The operation is done under a local anaesthetic with or without sedation, so it may take place either in the surgeon's operating office or in hospital. A surgical team is usually involved, working together using magnification: one person removes a strip from the scalp and sews up the wound, another trims away any excess fat from the graft and dices it into tiny plugs and yet another makes the holes ready to receive the micrografts.

Thousands of plugs can be transplanted like this – a bit like returfing the garden. Top surgeons have learned to take hair from areas where it's fine – such as the neck area – for the hairline. Slightly bigger plugs containing four or five hairs can be used a few rows back from the front to mimic the gradual thickening that occurs in a natural hairline.

The plugs of skin and cropped hair are held in place with a pressure bandage to try and curb bleeding. The scalp bleeds very easily and heavy bleeding is a common complication of hair surgery, so adrenaline is injected with the local anaesthetic to help control it.

Patients are told to keep the bandage on at night to protect the transplants and return next day when each transplant will have formed a scab. These last for 15 to 20 days and should be allowed to fall off naturally.

In fact, the transplanted hairs fall off at the same time as the scabs, but the live follicle is left behind in the scalp. It will start to produce hair after two or three months which will then grow at the normal rate of 1cm a month. You can shampoo gently after a week after regrowth starts but you must not use a hairbrush or comb near the grafts for two weeks.

The risks

There is always the risk that grafts will not take, leaving visible gaps. Several operations are required to fill in areas between previous grafts and achieve a natural look.

Micrografting works well for a receding hairline or for augmenting thin hair but it does not create a dense thicket – so careful styling is important – nor cover a completely bald pate.

The results of micrografting depend on the skill of the surgeon, who must make sure that implanted hair grows in the correct direction. Curly hair is most successful since it conceals the scalp better.

However, you must remember to take into account the likelihood of the baldness progressing as you grow older to avoid what happened to Sam Gould, a designer who's now 40.

'My hair started thinning when I was 24,' he says. 'I saw an ad for a clinic specialising in hair loss and when I went there

I was told that I could have plugs of hair moved from the back of my head to thicken up the front. I paid several thousand pounds to have it done. It was incredibly painful and there was a heck of a lot of bleeding. I had two sessions, as I recall, and that was it. I remember thinking that they hadn't looked after me at all well but the end result was OK and I was reasonably happy with it for ten years or so.'

The trouble was that Sam continued to go bald. As his fair hair got thinner, he was left with the plugs revealed – absurd tufts of hair and a pattern of little circular scars that showed up clearly on his exposed scalp.

'I looked ridiculous, so I went to another surgeon, who advised more plugs to fill in the bald surroundings. Well, after the first experience, I said no. I went to yet another surgeon and he advised electrolyisis to get rid of the plugs. That cost £500 and was painful but I was still left with a few wisps of hair and circular scars on top of my forehead.'

Sam has since consulted a fourth surgeon and is waiting for new treatment – dermabrasion (*see page 74*) to remove the top layers of skin and scar tissue on his scalp. He should, eventually, be left with the smooth, hairless dome he was so keen to avoid in his youth.

Alison Hudson, on the other hand, is pleased with her improved head of hair.

'I noticed that my hair was thinning quite badly at the temples so, as I was coming up to my fortieth birthday I decided to give myself a treat. I was working in Hollywood, so I went to the top guy. I had a strip removed from the back of my head and small plugs of five to seven hairs inserted in the temples.

'I had a local anaesthetic and sedation so I felt nothing for the two hours it took to have 60 implants. Afterwards, my head was bandaged and I was given painkillers and antibiotics. My head remained numb for a few hours and then I had a bit of a headache. Next day I went back to have the bandage removed and a light shampoo.

'The scabs soon came off and about ten weeks later tiny new hairs began to emerge, adding density exactly where it was needed. I was thrilled and, since then, I've had a couple more sessions to fill in where some of the plugs didn't take. I also use a dark cream on my scalp to hide the skin that still shows.'

Carried out by an expert, micrografting can be very successful. It's a relatively minor surgical procedure, though bleeding can be profuse and may continue after the operation, and there may be considerable pain. Disappointingly, not all plugs take. Micrografting cannot cover extensive areas of baldness and it should not be done on young men whose baldness will progress.

Artificial fibres made of nylon, on offer in parts of Europe, should never be implanted into the scalp. Artificial grafts often cause infection as the body does its best to reject the foreign material.

SCALP REDUCTION

Very bald men can have their bald patch made smaller by scalp reduction. This operation can only be done if the scalp is sufficiently mobile, which rules out older men, who generally have tight ones.

The surgeon simply cuts out the central area of baldness, usually under a local anaesthetic, and draws together and stitches the edges of skin, so that the hair-bearing areas of scalp are pulled right up, instantly covering more of the head with hair. It is sometimes carried out after tissue expansion (*see below*), which creates more hair-bearing skin.

The immediate result is an ugly scar, usually in the centre of the scalp, which takes seven to ten days to heal and may cause a decrease in scalp sensation. However, scalp reduction is usually done to deal with large areas of baldness and is often carried out prior to hair replacement surgery, when punch grafts can be used to conceal the scar.

TISSUE EXPANSION

The aim of tissue expansion is to create extra hair-bearing skin and, to do this, it involves the temporary insertion of silicone balloons under hair-bearing areas of the scalp. One larger crescent-shaped balloon, or two to three smaller balloons, are placed under the scalp and saline is injected into them, with top-ups at weekly intervals, to expand them. Over the course of three months, the head ends up bulging grotesquely.

The balloons are placed in such a way, adjacent to the bald patch, as to stretch the hairy areas of the scalp – just like pregnancy stretches the skin of the abdomen. When the balloons are removed, the bald area is cut out in a scalp reduction operation (*see above*) and the stretched skin manoeuvred over it, making sure that the blood supply to the skin flaps (*see page 198*) is maintained.

Tissue expansion does not create more hair, it simply stretches what you have so as to cover more of your head. It is the best way of covering large areas of baldness, but it is an expensive, lengthy and major procedure requiring considerable commitment on your part – it will keep you away from work for a couple of months while you look like an alien – and a properly trained plastic surgeon. (Tissue expansion is used by plastic surgeons treating burns patients and other victims of serious accidents.)

Two general anaesthetics will be required for two operations – insertion of the balloons and their removal three months later. Once the scalp starts to swell out, you will be reluctant to be seen. The swelling can be painful and the tissue expander can be expelled through the thinning skin, which can become infected.

Despite these drawbacks, tissue expansion can, in the right hands, be very successful.

SKIN FLAPS

Hair-bearing skin flaps are either created as a result of tissue expansion or they are cut out from the side or back of the scalp. The aim is to transfer the flaps to the front of the scalp while maintaining the flaps' supply of blood.

One ingenious technique is to take a long strip 15cm long and 2cm wide from each side of the scalp, with the base above the ear and close up the resulting wounds. The surgeon swivels the flaps through a 90-degree turn and drapes them in place into a prepared cut across the bald front of the scalp. This procedure creates two lumps at the base of each flap, where it is turned round. These can be removed later.

However, the hair in each flap is pointing backwards. So what the surgeon can do is to cut each one free and swap them round, reconnecting them on the opposite side of the head using microsurgery to join up the blood vessels. Now the hair is growing forwards in the right direction.

This is a major operation that is not widely practised in Britain. You're most likely to find it on offer in Japan and parts of South America.

Any surgery to the scalp runs the risk of severing nerves, which can leave you with changed sensation in the scalp and a painful feeling of pins and needles. In addition, wherever hair-bearing scalp is cut, hair will drop out – although it generally grows back three months later.

If you have thin or lightly coloured hair, then the scars from surgery to treat baldness will show up in certain situations, such as in the swimming pool or on a windy day.

HAIR WEAVING AND FUSION

The final option, of course, is disguise. The laurel wreath sported by Julius Caesar at the height of his powers was actually worn to conceal the imperial pate. Nowadays, it's more likely to be a toupée, although the toupée typically creates an unnatural hairline, especially when a man wistfully chooses a rich colour out of keeping with his own faded wisps.

If you're unhappy with your hairline, then you can get a surgeon to create one of your own (and a transitional zone of thicker hair) with punch grafts and then wear a partial hairpiece behind it over the balding spot.

Nowadays, the risk of a hairpiece blowing off in the wind

or under more private circumstances can be minimised by weaving the thatch into your remaining hair, or fusing in hair extensions to create a more successful and durable look.

Hair extensions can take up to three hours to have done. The microfibre extensions are plaited and heat-sealed on to existing hair, but they need to be replaced every eight to ten weeks, because they become more obvious as normal hair grows.

If you've got a hairline, but not enough hair, then you might opt for hair integration – a net-based hairpiece which allows your own hair to be drawn through the holes and blended with the false hair.

Cost: Micrografts, £8–10 each – you may need up to 400 grafts; scalp reduction, £1,200–1,500; tissue expansion, £4,000–5,000

Risks: bleeding; infection; loss of grafts; scars

Ideal age: depends on degree and area of baldness

Length of stay in hospital: day case

Anaesthetic: local

Other drugs: painkillers, antibiotics

Discomfort levels: moderate to high

Time before the signs of surgery disappear: 4 months

Length of time results last: permanent

CHAPTER FOURTEEN

How to Find a Surgeon,

WHAT TO ASK WHEN YOU'VE FOUND ONE

AND WHAT TO DO IF THINGS GO WRONG

Y ou've decided to take the plunge, but you don't know
how to find a reputable cosmetic surgeon. It's a
common problem and there's no easy answer.

Cosmetic surgery is largely unregulated in Britain.
Anyone who has graduated from medical school can hang
up a sign and practise privately as a cosmetic surgeon.
There's now some official training for it – but it's an art
rather than a science and it's mostly learned from obser-
vation and practice. So how do you distinguish a good
surgeon from a cowboy?

First, some history. Since the 1939–45 war, when many
badly burned fighter pilots were successfully patched up,
Britain has enjoyed a fine reputation for plastic reconstructive surgery.

There are now around 150 plastic surgeons in Britain,
who are trained over many years to carry out reconstructive
surgery under the NHS on patients injured in accidents, deformed from birth or disfigured by burns or cancer. The
word plastic comes from the Greek and means to mould.

Many of these plastic surgeons also practise cosmetic
surgery privately, but some may be relatively inexperienced
because less and less cosmetic work is done on the NHS.

The NHS gives priority to reconstructive surgery for people disfigured by disease or injury, although certain cosmetic procedures – including ear-pinning and breast reduction – are still allowed.

The surgeon must, however, be convinced that surgery will relieve real psychological distress caused by the offending feature before you can have it done on the NHS. Then, even if you find an NHS plastic surgeon sympathetic to your cause, the waiting list for a cosmetic operation may be long and you cannot choose who does it.

So you're likely to want to go privately, which means you'll be embarking on major and costly surgery. An inexperienced surgeon may disappoint you, or even scar you. There's no guarantee and no real qualification of expertise.

The usual advice is to ask your GP – and any other doctors if you happen to know them – for the names of surgeons who specialise in the sort of operation you want. Your GP should know the reputable cosmetic surgeons in the locality. More than one name means more choice. Look out for a name which gets mentioned by doctors more than once.

Some surgeons want the GP to write them a referral letter. And if you already have the name of a surgeon you would like to see, then your GP can arrange an appointment. If your GP is unhelpful or unsympathetic, consult another. You have a perfect right to gain access to a cosmetic surgeon if you want.

There is no excuse for your GP to be vague. Hospitals provide them with a list of their surgeons and the professional organisations which represent cosmetic surgeons have sent a register of their members to every GP in the country. This has been done specifically to help point patients in the right direction.

But you don't have to approach your GP at all. You can

contact a surgeon directly yourself, if you have a name, although surgeons often prefer a traditional referral. Some people are shy about approaching their busy GP about something to do with their appearance. They may fear ridicule. They may not know their GP very well and shrink from discussing something so personal. Or they may know their GP socially. They may live in a small community and not wish to risk friends knowing that they seek cosmetic surgery.

So the other good way of finding a surgeon's name is through personal recommendation.

If you know anyone who's had cosmetic surgery – and it's more common than you might think – and you are impressed with the result, then ask them who did it.

Beauty therapists and hairdressers come into contact with a lot of people who may have had cosmetic surgery. So ask them and ask your friends if they know anyone who's had it.

It's obviously most helpful if you can talk to someone who's had the same operation as the one that you want. But of course the trouble in Britain is that most people who have cosmetic surgery keep quiet about it. So then what?

Private clinics

Look through the back pages of any glossy magazine or even *Yellow Pages* and you'll find advertisements for clinics promising you an improved face or body via cosmetic surgery. Individual doctors are strictly prohibited from advertising their services but private clinics are allowed to advertise. However, some clinics have been reprimanded by the Advertising Standards Authority for printing misleading information.

Private clinics are attractive to anyone seeking anonymity, but it is important to remember that they are strictly commercial. A common complaint is that, when you arrive, you are often met by a representative who immediately tries to sell you an operation before you've even had a chance to talk to a surgeon. Then, when you do, there's no way of assessing his or her competence. The skill of these clinic surgeons varies enormously. Some can be highly recommended, others not at all.

You may also run across some so-called surgical advisors. These are self-appointed people, usually women who may have had cosmetic surgery, who have set up advisory agencies. Some may be truly independent but others have direct financial links with particular clinics or surgeons.

So how do you find out whether a surgeon is any good? You can look at the letters after their name. But almost all surgeons have the letters FRCS after their name. These stand for Fellow of the Royal College of Surgeons (of England, Edinburgh, Glasgow or Ireland) and all they mean is that the surgeon has received a basic training in general surgery early in his or her career. The letters FRCS do not mean that the surgeon has any specific training in plastic or cosmetic surgery.

Plastic surgeons trained in this country, however, have to pass an exam in plastic surgery that includes an exam in aesthetic (cosmetic) surgery and includes six years' training in NHS plastic surgery as part of an approved specialist training. These surgeons can be recognised by the letters FRCS (T).

The General Medical Council (GMC), which is the governing body of all doctors, holds lists of specialist trained surgeons, including a list of plastic surgeons. So if you want to know if your surgeon is a specialist ring the GMC (0171 580 7642) and ask if his or her name is on the specialist register. Increasingly, surgeons who have trained in Europe are allowed to practise in this country, but they will not be on this list unless they have completed specialist plastic surgery training.

Organisations to contact

Plastic surgeons who carry out cosmetic work usually belong to an association which is involved in training and education. The British Association of Aesthetic Plastic Surgeons (BAAPS) has 140 members, all of whom are, or have been, consultant plastic surgeons in the NHS and are members of the British Association of Plastic Surgeons (BAPS), which is concerned with NHS reconstructive surgery. They are all on the GMC specialist list. BAAPS has been approved by the Royal College of Surgeons as the official organisation to educate and train cosmetic surgeons and it is part of the International Society of Aesthetic Plastic Surgery.

The BAAPS secretary says that she has been receiving 40 requests a day for information about cosmetic surgery. If you send her a large stamped (first class) addressed envelope, she will send you a list of members and also further information about different surgical procedures.

There is also a rival group, the British Association of Cosmetic Surgeons (BACS), which was set up in 1979 by a group of surgeons who found they were doing a lot of cosmetic work. BACS has a smaller membership and represents many of the surgeons working for private clinics or hospitals that advertise directly to the public.

To complicate matters further, there are also some independent cosmetic surgeons, including some ear, nose and throat surgeons and some ophthalmic surgeons who carry out cosmetic nose, ear or eyelid operations (who may be on the GMC specialist list for their speciality) who belong to neither BAPS, BAAPS nor BACS.

There is considerable hostility between the BAPS/BAAPS and BACS factions. It is fair to say that there are some good and some not so good surgeons in both camps.

Orthodox plastic and reconstructive surgeons may be suspicious of BACS members and independent cosmetic surgeons because they have not undergone years of intensive training in NHS reconstructive work. BACS members and some of the independent surgeons, on the other hand, tend to believe that their cosmetic work is superior to that of plastic surgeons because they spend all their time doing it and are therefore very practised.

Your first consultation with a surgeon should cost between £35 and £75, although some surgeons give their initial consultations free. This is the most important sum of money that you will pay out because the surgeon will decide at this consultation whether he or she can fulfil your expectations and you will be assessing whether he or she is the surgeon you want to operate on you.

It's definitely worth talking to more than one surgeon, although you may resent spending this amount of money on window shopping. It is important to find out what different surgeons can offer you and which is technically most competent and experienced at the kind of operation you seek.

WHAT YOU NEED TO KNOW

Ask how many years experience the surgeon has and how many similar operations he performs each week. Do not be fobbed off with generalisations. You are entitled to an honest and truthful answer. Some cosmetic surgeons cover a range of procedures while others specialise in particular operations. You don't really want to have your nose done by someone who's best at doing breasts.

You need to feel comfortable with him or her and feel that you can trust him or her. You also need to be sure that you and the surgeon are in agreement about what you hope to achieve. We all have our own views on beauty and a cosmetic surgeon may have strong views that do not match yours or that you feel are wrong for you. You will only find all this out through having a long chat.

You must be able to set out exactly what it is you seek to change. The surgeon needs to know precisely what bothers you. Then he or she can offer an opinion as to whether surgery can achieve the change you desire and what it would involve – in terms of money, time and discomfort.

The surgeon will ask you about your medical history and will want to know why you want surgery. So you want to feel relaxed about telling him your hang-ups.

You want to hear all about preparing for surgery; the operation itself and how long it takes; what kind of anaesthesia will be used; whether you will have to stay in hospital; how long you can expect to be in pain, bruised and swollen; when stitches will be removed; the healing process; scarring; total recovery time; and how long the results will last. Many surgeons provide printed material with details of the various operations for you to take away.

Ask whether there are any before and after photographs of the kind of surgery you want. But remember that a surgeon will probably show you his or her best work – people look glamorous and cheerful in 'after' photographs, compared with them looking drab and miserable in 'before' photographs. And photographs of other people's results are no guarantee of what you might expect because they take no account of factors, such as skin elasticity and scar healing, which make your outcome unique. You might want to ask the surgeon to draw (if applicable) the expected result of the operation. Computer imaging may be exciting, but it is no guarantee of your outcome.

You must make sure that the person you're talking to is the person who will carry out the surgery. And be sure that you have a second consultation before you consent to an operation. It is well known that people only take in a third of what they hear when they consult a doctor.

Look around the surgeon's consulting rooms and talk to the nurse and secretary. These people will probably be important in looking after you if you decide to have surgery.

Above all, it's very important that you are told in detail about the risks involved. Any surgeon who does not mention the possible adverse effects of surgery should be viewed with suspicion. And you also need to know how much it is all going to cost, including the price of additional surgery if complications arise.

There is no insurance that you can take out to cover you if an operation should go wrong and you have to go back into hospital. But most surgeons will belong to one of three organisations – the Medical Defence Union, the Medical Protection Society or the Medical and Dental Defence Union of Scotland – which provide them with indemnity against the results of legal actions by patients unhappy about their treatment. It is a cause for concern if they don't belong to one of these three organisations. A handful of doctors have had so many legal actions made against them for professional

negligence or other matters that none of these three organisations will cover them, so they are covered instead by another
insurance company.

So another question you might legitimately ask a cosmetic
surgeon would be about his insurance arrangements with
regard to cover against a legal claim.

Don't be afraid to ask questions – it's the only way to get
any answers. The best way is to make a list of everything
you want to find out and take it to the consultation. You
might even like to take notes while you're there.

He or she should answer all your questions in language
that you understand and should not put any pressure on you
to have a particular operation. He or she should also accept
that you will want to consult another surgeon in order to
compare notes.

'I went to see three separate surgeons,' says Louise
Warner, a nurse who's 45 and wanted her eyes done. 'I paid
£35 to one, £50 to another and nothing to the third. They
all seemed competent and I found it hard to make up my
mind. In the end I simply chose the one I liked best – the
other two were just a little too casual for my liking. And I
was very happy with my choice.'

WHAT IF IT ALL GOES WRONG?

Undoubtedly, there are some people who have been left injured
or disfigured by cosmetic surgery that has gone wrong. But the
vast majority are very happy with their surgery.

If you feel that your operation has gone wrong, how do
you set about getting redress? The first step is a practical
one: go back and tell your surgeon that you are not happy

with the result. A reasonable surgeon will often perform a second operation to correct the fault with no additional surgeon's fee – but you still may have to pay for hospital accommodation,

However, it may be that you no longer feel confident in his or her work. In this case, you will want a second opinion which your surgeon may arrange for you, or you may wish to find someone for yourself. If your surgeon refers you to a colleague, you need to establish first of all who will pay for the consultation and for any subsequent surgery (occasionally two surgeons may have an arrangement to help each other out in such situations).

Remember that no secondary surgery can be carried out until scars have softened – this is usually at least a year after your first operation.

But you may prefer to take legal action. You can only sue a surgeon for negligence or assault and battery. A surgeon is negligent if he or she falls below an accepted standard of advice, operative performance and/or aftercare. Assault and battery is if a surgeon carries out a procedure which you haven't agreed to. This means the surgeon *must* secure the patient's *informed consent*. Informed consent means explaining to you in such a way that you understand the operative procedure, the recovery, the result and the possible complications. You will be asked to sign a piece of paper before the operation agreeing that all of this has been explained to you. This consent form is not legally binding on either side.

Suppose, for instance, you had a breast reduction and a nipple died. If the surgeon did not tell you that this might happen at one of the consultations, then you might be able to sue him because you did not give informed consent.

If you were told about this, you cannot sue the surgeon for negligence because nipple loss is a recognised complication of breast reduction.

Taking legal action

If you do decide to take legal action, then your first port of call should be an organisation called Action for Victims of Medical Accidents (1 London Road, Forest Hill, London SE23 3TP, tel: 0181 291 2793) which will point you in the direction of a solicitor who specialises in medical cases.

If you have a legitimate complaint, then you stand a good chance of a financial settlement in your favour. However, taking legal action is always a lottery, and if you are not entitled to legal aid, the cost of bringing an action may be prohibitive.

Normally, you have to issue proceedings for a claim within three years of the date of surgery. The solicitor will advise you at each step of the way along the lengthy process of making a claim. Your medical notes will be examined regarding the advice you received as to the risks of surgery and the technique used. If it appears that your complaint is well founded, then the opinion of an independent surgeon will be sought.

Most valid claims are settled out of court, partly because the surgeon will want to avoid any lurid publicity which often accompanies a court case. The amount of money obtained in a settlement is variable and depends on a number of factors that vary from case to case, even when they appear very similar.

However, legal action is a lottery. If you are unsuccessful in your claim and you are not on legal aid, you run the risk of having to pay not only your own costs of bringing the action but also the surgeon's costs of defending.

So be sure to think through all the possible results – good and bad – of having cosmetic surgery before you decide to have that operation. Even the best cosmetic surgeons have patients who are disappointed afterwards. There are simply no guarantees. But you will be happy so long as the benefits of having a cosmetic operation outweigh the risks.

COMMON CONCERNS AND WHAT CAN BE DONE ABOUT THEM

Worries	Treatments
All-over facial sagging	face-lift
Vertical frown lines	botulinum toxin, collagen injections, brow-lift
Horizontal forehead lines	botulinum toxin, brow-lift
Crow's feet	Retin A cream, botulinum toxin, laser resurfacing
Acne pits	surgery, dermabrasion, laser resurfacing, collagen injections
Eyelid hoods/bags	eyelid surgery
Nose-to-mouth grooves	SMAS face-lift
Lipstick lines	dermabrasion, chemical peel, laser resurfacing
Neck rings	peel, SMAS face-lift
Spider veins	sclerotherapy, laser treatment
Liver spots	laser treatment, cryo surgery
Drooping breasts	mastopexy and/or implants
Small breasts	implants
Large breasts	breast reduction
Flabby arms	arm reduction
Floppy belly	tummy tuck
Bulging thighs/hips	liposuction
Cellulite	liposuction
Stretch marks	no treatment
Ageing hands	no treatment

Useful Addresses

British Association of Aesthetic Plastic Surgeons at the Royal College of Surgeons (BAAPS)
35 Lincoln's Inn Fields
London WC2A 3PN

Tel: 0171 405 2234

A list of fully accredited cosmetic plastic surgeons is available from the BAAPS office by sending a large, stamped, first class, self-addressed envelope to the address above. If you also mention the specific procedure you seek, they will enclose the appropriate factsheet.

British Association of Cosmetic Surgeons (BACS)
17 Harley Street
London W1N 1DA

Tel: 0171 323 5728
Fax: 01590 624 114

A list of members and any other information you may require is available from this association by contacting the association at the above address.

British Association of Plastic Surgeons at the Royal College of Surgeons (BAPS)
35-43 Lincoln's Inn Fields
London WC2A 3PN

Tel: 0171 831 5161/2
Fax: 0171 831 4041

The Association is concerned with burns and reconstructive surgery and does not release its list of members to the general public or outside organisations.

International Society of Aesthetic Plastic Surgery (ISAPS)
c/o David Harris MS FRCS
British National Secretary, ISAPS
Nuffield Hospital
Derriford Road
Plymouth PL6 8BG

Tel: 01752 707 345
Fax: 01752 778 421

The British membership of ISAPS is relatively small and all members are also BAAPS members.

Index